Burn Fat, Build Muscle

Two Books Bundle: Burn Fat Fast: Ridiculously Effective Flab Busting Secrets Revealed
&
Strength Training Program 101: Build Muscle And Burn Fat...

In Less Than 3 Hours Per Week

By

Marc McLean

©Copyright 2017

By Marc McLean – All rights reserved

Author's Legal Disclaimer

This book is solely for informational and educational purposes and is not medical advice. Please consult a medical or health professional before you begin any new exercise, nutrition or supplementation program, or if you have questions about your health.

The information in this book is not a prescription and does not make any claim about health improvements, or any difference to your health in its own right. There are many elements to good health.

Any use of the information within this book is at the reader's discretion and risk. The author cannot be held responsible for any loss, claim or damage arising out of the use, or misuse, of the suggestions made, the failure to take medical advice, or for any related material from third party sources. No part of this publication shall be reproduced, transmitted, or sold in any form without the prior written consent of the author.

All trademarks and registered trademarks appearing in this digital book are the property of their respective owners.

Table of Contents

Burn Fat Fast: Ridiculously Effective Flab Busting Secrets Revealed 1

Introduction 2

Part One: It's Not Just What You Eat… 5

    Say Goodbye To That Damn, Stubborn, Annoying, Lingering Fat… 6

    Introducing Intermittent Fasting 9

    It's As Simple As Skipping Breakfast 11

    Success Stories 13

    Learning From The Experts 15

Part Two: Exercise Like A Boss 17

    Lift Weights (Heavy Only Please) 18

    How Often - And How Long - Should You Be Training For? 21

    The Fat Loss Fast Lane 23

    Eight Reasons Why You Should Be Sprinting 24

    Rapid Steps To Sprint Success 29

    Tabata Training 33

Part Three: No Nonsense Nutrition 35

    Sugar Ain't So Sweet 36

    Eating Clean Made Simple 38

    Why Energy Drinks Are To Be Avoided 42

    Keeping Your Calories In Check 45

    Delay Your Post-Workout Shake 48

    One Positive Habit Per Week 50

Part Four: Fat Burning Hacks 54
   Training In The Morning On An Empty Stomach 55
   Supercharge Your Workouts With Black Coffee 57
   Give Green Tea The Green Light 60
   The Magic Of Lemon Water 62
Conclusion 66

Strength Training Program 101: Build Muscle & Burn Fat In Less Than 3 Hours Per Week 71

Introduction 72
Chapter 1: Cutting Out the Confusion 78
Chapter 2: Preparation and Goal Setting For Maximum Results 88
Chapter 3: The Secret To Staying On Track 100
Chapter 4: Building Muscle and Burning Fat Through Compound Exercises 105
Chapter 5: Compound Exercises: Bigger Movements, Better Results 113
Chapter 6: Muscle Isolation Moves 125
Chapter 7: How To Create Your Own Training Plans .. 140
Chapter 8: 9 Essential Ingredients To Better Nutrition 150
Chapter 9: 10 Reasons You've Not Been Building Muscle And Losing Fat 157
Conclusion 166
About the author 173

Burn Fat Fast:

Ridiculously Effective Flab Busting Secrets Revealed

Introduction

Burning bodyfat is one of the easiest things in the world to do…

Yes easy. Yet so many people make such hard work of it. Sweating through boring exercise sessions that they don't really enjoy. Making themselves miserable eating salads, low fat foods and struggling like hell resisting their favourite treats.

Then they step on the scales a few weeks later, see that they've barely lost a single pound, and then lose the plot. Frustration reaches boiling point and there's only one thing for it…

Order a Chinese takeaway, get that half eaten tub of ice cream out the freezer, head to the shop and buy 17 bars of chocolate.

Does any of this sound even slightly familiar to you? Most of us who are less than happy with the shape we're in end up on the same merry-go-round of training/dieting > getting pissed off at the lack of results > going on a junk food bender > ending up back at square one.

It doesn't have to be that way. This book is your saviour! Follow the advice in the following chapters and you'll be able to turn your body into a fat burning machine.

I'll say it again: burning fat and staying lean is actually easy. It's just that most men and women go the wrong way about it.

Exercising ineffectively. Trying to eat healthily but doing so in an unhealthy way by following fad diets, or nutrition plans that are just way too complicated. The usual end result is failure simply because it's too difficult to maintain in the long run.

Fact is: nutrition accounts for about 70% of your success when it comes to achieving your health and fitness goals. If you're following an extreme diet or super strict nutrition plan then it's going to end in disaster as some point. Sure, you might get some results at first but you'll eventually lose willpower (and possibly the will to live!) and will inevitably return to old habits and pile the weight back on again.

What this book preaches is not only healthy eating, but a *healthy way of eating* that is sensible, do-able and manageable. You won't wanna punch me in the face after a week of following my nutritional advice. Notice that I say nutritional advice; we don't do 'diets' around here. Diets are unnatural, unnecessary and the results they bring are usually only temporary.

Here's more good news: you'll still be able to eat your favourite foods (without going mental) and lose weight. Everything in moderation is acceptable because the strategies in this book will elevate your metabolism levels (which equals fat burned) and will also force your body to use up its fat stores (…yes, even more fat incinerated).

How To Burn Fat Fast is split into four sections covering meal timing, exercise, nutrition, and fat burning hacks. These are the key areas for your success and each of them has ultra effective strategies that have a proven track record for creating fine, lean human specimens!

Combine all of the strategies included in these chapters and it's virtually impossible not to lose weight fast. If you do all of the above consistently, I'm pretty confident you'll be amazed at your body transformation. It doesn't matter how many times you've failed in the past, how overweight you are, or whether you're a man or woman. These tactics will blitz your bodyfat. I've witnessed it time and again with personal training clients, and friends and family who hound me for training/nutritional advice to lose fat.

The best part? It's not as hard as you think. You can potentially see a quick shift in your weight within the first week simply by following the ultra effective meal timing advice in chapter one. It might take a bit longer, along with combining the exercise strategies in part two, and the fat burning hacks in part four.

This is simply because we're all different. Our bodies are all various shapes and sizes, we have different metabolic rates, some readers are younger and more physically able than others. These factors all play a part in how quickly your bodyfat levels drop and your body shape changes. But you CAN do it.

Of course, it takes action, commitment and consistency from you too. You're more than capable of managing everything I describe in this book…and becoming a leaner, healthier, better version of yourself!

Part One

It's Not Just What You Eat…

Say Goodbye To That Damn, Stubborn, Annoying, Lingering Fat…

I had no idea so many guys struggled shifting the flab from their bellies. No clue that countless women think they are fat. And I didn't realise that so many people were doing so many ineffective things to try and get in shape.

People always tell me, "it's easy for you to say, you've always been slim." True - the main reason I kick-started my obsession with weight training and health and fitness in general back in 1998 was because I was so skinny. I hated being built like a rake and this created personal body image issues that most overweight people have too.

So I'm afraid I simply haven't got an amazing personal success story of how I went from fatboy to slimshady in a matter of weeks. Or shocking before and after pictures to prove it. Instead, I'll share several stories of clients, friends and family who have achieved just that - by following my training, nutrition and lifestyle advice. That very same advice is included in this book so you can finally hit your own health and fitness goals, and be proud of the new you.

When I set up my online personal training business last year I ran a Facebook advert to get clients for my men's body transformation programme. I asked people to fill in a questionnaire about their fitness goals and was expecting guys to be asking me to show them "how to build bigger biceps", "gain muscle mass", or simply learn how to create bigger, stronger bodies.

The responses I got surprised me. Out of nearly 50 guys from around the UK, more than half said their main goal was to lose weight or get rid of their belly fat. Below are some of their comments (I've not included their full names or locations because I don't have their permission).

David: "While I've achieved a slimmer physique, there is still some flab around my waist and I cannot develop visible muscle or a six pack."

Colin: "I want to bring my stomach in and lose weight overall."

Sid: "I'd like to lose weight for my high cholesterol, aswell as to be able to wear clothes I've not been able to wear for a while."

Spencer: "The biggest challenge is getting rid of the fat on my body. I can never lose it properly no matter what I try. I lose a bit then plateau and cannot break through to lose the gut where the majority of fat seems to sit."

Richard: "My problem is shedding fat around the love handles. It is going gradually but it just takes ages!"

Can you relate to any of these problems? If you're a woman it may be that you're desperate to lose weight from your hips, thighs or butt as these are lower body regions where females naturally store more bodyfat. For guys, the problem areas are primarily the upper body and belly.

I also asked the guys about their current weekly training regime and what their diet was like. You'd think that a chunk of them just didn't exercise enough but some of these guys were exercising 4 or 5 days per week, and their diets didn't seem too unhealthy (based on what they told me).

Why then were they all facing the same stumbling blocks? Why could they just not shift that damn, stubborn, annoying, lingering fat?

Firstly, how many days you train or how long you exercise for is not quite as important. The type of exercise - and the intensity of it - is what separates the mediocre results from the marvellous.

Secondly, these people had no clue about the calories they were taking in and expending each day. Calories are important; and if the input is more than the output consistently then you're inevitably going to put on weight. Don't worry, I'm not expecting you to start counting calories every time you eat - that would just be ridiculous. However, it's important you have a rough idea of your daily calorie intake and I'm going to share with you a tactic that makes this so easy to track.

Thirdly, none of these guys were implementing the full range of fat burning hacks that I reveal in Part Four.

And finally, not one of them had employed - or even heard of - what I consider the single most effective tactic for stripping bodyfat (while maintaining lean muscle). This is the number one piece of advice I give to men and women looking to burn fat and develop a leaner body. Some of my clients have seen some outstanding results with it. It's backed by solid science, it has numerous other health benefits, and it's much easier to implement than hopping about from one crazy fad diet to another.

I'm talking about…intermittent fasting.

Introducing Intermittent Fasting

What was your first reaction when you read "intermittent fasting" on the previous page?

Did the voice in your head say something like: "Fuck this, I'm not fasting…I'm not really into starving!"

Unless you've already heard about intermittent fasting and are clued-up on how it works, then that's the kind of response I get from most people when I first mention those words. They might not say it, but I can see from the reaction on their faces that the word "fasting" has put the fear into them.

I'm going to give a simple explanation about how it works, how I first came across it five or six years ago, and I'll also serve up a few stories of personal training clients and friends who've experienced amazing results with intermittent fasting.

First, let's get a few things straight.

Intermittent fasting is NOT:

- Some sort of diet plan, it simply involves adjusting the time you eat your meals.

- Hard to stick with, in fact it's much easier than following any fad diet.

- Dangerous or unhealthy in any way, in fact it has numerous health benefits.

- Reliant on willpower, it's just a case of your body adjusting to a new eating schedule.

Intermittent fasting IS:

- An effective way of burning fat without going on a super restrictive diet.

- A more natural way of eating which harks back to the 'hunter gatherer' days of our ancestors.

- Beneficial for your digestive system as gives it a rest from breaking down large volumes of food often.

- Backed by science as an effective way of regenerating your cells and boosting your immune system.

How Intermittent Fasting Works

So what is intermittent fasting? It means having an extended break between your meals in order to trigger a natural fat burning response in your body. Our body builds up glycogen stores from the food we eat and this is our main source of energy for our activities and to get through the day.

When we go for long breaks without food our glycogen bank run out - and our body is forced to turn to bodyfat for energy.

How long is that break without food? Generally a period of 14-18 hours. Once you get beyond the 14 hour mark of no food supply, the body will eat into fat stores for energy. As you get nearer the 18 hour mark, more and more coal is being added to your body's fat burning fire.

I know what you're thinking…"how the hell am I going to last without food for 14 hours or more?" That may sound like torture at first, but it's easier than you think because this period also takes into account your sleeping hours.

When we're sleeping we're effectively fasting for 8 hours, or however long you're snoozing. All we have to do next is extend that by another six hours and we're in the fat burning zone.

It's As Simple As Skipping Breakfast

You can achieve your intermittent fasting goal simply by skipping breakfast. All you have to do is ensure there's at least a 14 hour gap between your last meal in the evening and your first meal the following day.

It's flexible and here's how it can play out easily in various ways…

Scenario 1: You finish eating dinner with the family at 8pm, go to bed a few hours later, and then head to work without eating breakfast. But you're a clever dude and have packed some food on-the-go in your bag and whip them out in the office at 11am. So, 8pm-11am is a break of 15 hours - job done!

Scenario 2: You get in from work late and dinner has basically become supper as you're now finishing it at 9.30pm. No sweat because you skip breakfast the following day and don't eat lunch until 12noon. That's an intermittent fasting period of 14.5 hours - job done!

Scenario 3: It's 10am and you're feeling really hungry. You remember that the last time you ate yesterday was around 6pm…so that means there's already a 16 hour intermittent fasting period. You're good to go.

I think you get the picture. The times you eat can be flexible and can fit around your life. It's basically just a case of making sure there's a gap of at least 14 hours between your last meal your first meal today and your last meal yesterday.

You may still not be 100% sold on the idea, thinking it's going to be too difficult to maintain. Trust me, it's easier than you think - and definitely much easier than following extreme diets where various foods are completely banned.

Intermittent fasting simply focuses on the *timing* of your meals, rather than the *foods included* in your meals. No foods are banned and it certainly gives you a bit more freedom when it comes to your daily food choices. That being said, I don't recommend eating a multi-pack of Mars bars the minute you exceed the 14 hour mark of your fast. That's not exactly gonna work.

I'll go into nutrition and the types of foods you should be eating - and avoiding - in Part Three. I'm just trying to make the point that intermittent fasting is a completely new approach to losing weight and keeping it off.

If you've tried all sorts of diets to burn fat and got nowhere, this single tactic might well be the answer to your prayers. I say that confidently because I've seen it work wonders with clients who struggled big time with their weight.

While I've always been a naturally slimmer guy who finds it hard to gain weight, I also follow intermittent fasting because it keeps my bodyfat levels low effortlessly. I eat a clean diet Monday-Friday and train hard 3-4 days per week, but at the weekend I eat junk food that would otherwise result in a flabby belly. It never happens - because intermittent fasting (and my heavy weight training regime) compensates and keeps me in great shape.

Success Stories

I got a Facebook private message from Colin McIntyre - a guy I hadn't heard from in years - in November 2016. He wrote: "Are you still doing personal training? I'd really like you to help me get into shape?"

Here's my disclaimer upfront - Colin is my cousin, so he's obviously going to say nothing but good things about the help I gave him! But I'm relaying his story here because I think it's one that many readers will be able to relate to.

Colin's a married dad-of-two, who works long hours, and admitted that maintaining a healthy diet was always his biggest struggle. He'd reached his heaviest ever weight and was desperate to get rid of his overhanging belly.

First, we swapped his running for lifting heavy weights. Next, he was expecting a strict, rigid meal plan from me. That's not exactly how it worked out.

Rather than ban all sorts of foods and insist that Colin lives on chicken and steamed broccoli most of the week, I simply instructed him to skip breakfast every day and following some foundational nutritional advice (as described later in Part Three).

Here's what happened…

"For years I used to go out running for miles to try and get in decent shape," said Colin. "It was usually the same route, it was usually boring as hell, and I was lucky if I lost one, maybe two pounds.

"I'd just get fed up after 2-3 weeks and go back to eating junk food again. After joining Marc's programme and doing the intermittent fasting I dropped 15lbs in the first month alone.

"Everyone could see the difference in me. My boss had been off work for 6 weeks and when he came back the first thing he said to me was, 'man, you've lost some weight!'

"I went through the Christmas and New Year period afterwards expecting to gain some weight again but it stayed at the same level. I was really surprised at that."

Intermittent fasting was undoubtedly a big factor in Colin's success as diet was the big problem area for him, but combining this with my specific weight training programme supercharged his results. (We move onto the brilliant fat-burning benefits of lifting weights in Part Two).

Chris Hannan signed up to my body transformation programme in March this year because he had a holiday coming up. He'd also piled on the weight and wanted to burn fat fast before hitting the beach.

"My holiday is in a fortnight…do you think I can lose some weight by then?", he said.

He didn't exactly give me much time to work a miracle, but I was confident intermittent fasting would deliver surprising results. Chris was simply advised to skip breakfast, cut his calories slightly, lift weights three times per week, and limit sugar/junk foods.

The result? He lost 10lbs in 10 days, more than he expected before his holiday. As I've just mentioned, there were several changes to Chris' lifestyle in terms of nutrition and training, but intermittent fasting was undoubtedly the most effective element.

Learning From The Experts

Considering how effective it is and how easy it is to follow, I'm surprised the intermittent fasting phenomenon isn't more widespread. The word is slowly getting out there and I've recently spoken to a few gym instructors who have educated themselves on its benefits and are passing the message on.

I first came across the fasting approach about five or six years ago after buying the book 'The Warrior Die't by Ori Hofmekler. Author of several health and fitness/sports nutrition books and founder of Defense Nutrition, Ori's knowledge of sports science and how the human body works is on a different planet.

The premise of The Warrior Diet is that we fast during the day - and feast at night. He argues that this is how we as humans are biologically engineered to survive because in caveman days humans would often spend many hours during the day hunting for food, and then would eat their 'catch' by the fire at night.

Ori explains how this approach of fasting for a long period and feasting during a smaller window ramps up fat burning and helps create a leaner, more athletic body. Big name athletes who follow The Warrior Diet include former women's world UFC champion Ronda Rousey and kettlebell expert Pavel Tsatsouline. Now aged 65, Ori is in better shape than most guys in their 20's.

That was my first introduction to the concept of intermittent fasting, and I was completely sold on it after reading the book 'Eat Stop Eat' by Brad Pilon. While researching the book, nutritional expert Brad reviewed hundreds of scientific papers and reviews into the effects of intermittent fasting.

There had been some claims by sceptics and critics that fasting for extended periods could cause metabolic damage or lead to health issues in the long term.

In the book, Brad writes: "Almost all of the scientific research I reviewed provided evidence in direct opposition to the misinformation found in diet books and on the internet. I found very convincing evidence that supports the use of short term fasting as an effective weight loss tool.

"This included research on the effect that fasting has on your memory and cognitive abilities, your metabolism and muscle, and the effect that fasting has on exercise and exercise performance."

How Long Should You Fast?

If you want to delve deeper into the workings of intermittent fasting, or the science behind it, then I'd highly recommend Brad's book Eat Stop Eat. He's the main man when it comes to this particular area and I've yet to read a better book on this single topic.

Are you ready to give it a go (and I highly recommend you do) but are not sure how long you should be fasting for? 14 hours, 15…18?

There's no one definitive answer because how quickly we burn fat depends on various factors including our age, activity level, metabolic rate etc. Fourteen hours is typically the minimum period before fat burning really begins to kick in, and for me personally the sweet spot is 14-16 hours.

For those who are very overweight or want to have the best chance of burning fat fastest, then I'd aim for 16-18 hours between your first meal of the day and last meal the previous day.

I've seen intermittent fasting work wonders. I'm certain it can do the same for you.

Part Two

Exercise Like A Boss

Lift Weights (Heavy Only Please)

I'm always banging on about lifting weights to anyone that'll listen…

My 93-year-old neighbour. The woman that served me in Aldi yesterday. Random folk I see looking bored to tears on the treadmill. That's because most people have got the wrong idea about weight training.

It's NOT all about building muscle…

It's not just for fitter, stronger, younger people…

Or guys wearing muscle vests and make loud grunting noises in the gym.

Weight training/strength training is highly effective for burning fat - much more so than standard cardio exercise. For some reason, many people still think that cardio is for fat loss and weight training is for muscle gain. Like it's that black and white.

I was speaking to a friend of a friend in the gym last week who doing bench presses, barbell biceps curls and a couple of other really effective weight training exercises. But then he cut his weights session short to head for the cardio machines.

He told me: "I'm enjoying lifting some weights and I'm feeling stronger but I'm doing 30 minutes of cardio next because I need to lose this flab around my belly. I just can't seem to shift it."

His split exercise approach - doing a half-hearted weights session and half-assed cardio workout - was clearly one of the main problems.

Same thing happened a few days later when I bumped into an old schoolmate in the gym. He was looking for advice to get in shape. I asked him what his main goals were and what he'd been doing up until now to try and achieve them.

He said: "I want to add more muscle up top, in my chest area, shoulders and arms. I've been doing weight training nearly every day the past two weeks.

"I'm not getting any younger and I've got a bit of a pot belly these days, so I'm also playing five-a-side football and doing sit-ups at home."

Another flawed approach for two reasons. One - he was lifting weights too frequently which will hamper results and lead to burnout in the long run. A better approach is to give the body roughly around 48 hours to recover if you're training properly with heavy weights at the right intensity.

Secondly, he'd also bought into the notion that cardio exercise and a ton of sit-ups will get rid of his bulging belly. Afraid not.

Weight Training Develops Lean Muscle AND Burns Bodyfat

The reality is that cardio burns some calories, can help you lose some fat (in an inefficient way), and it does zilch for muscle tone.

Meanwhile, weight training keeps calories burning long after you stop training. Studies have shown that heavy resistance training can keep metabolism levels elevated up to 24 hours after exercise. With standard cardio training this 'after-burn' period is much shorter. Weight training also sparks muscle development and remodelling through a process called hypertrophy (aka muscle tissue growth). How do you reach hypertrophy effectively? By lifting heavy weights and pushing yourself hard in the gym.

I'm a huge fan of 'compound exercises' and these are the moves that make up the majority of my workouts and the training plans of my online PT clients. I'm talking about the big moves that have been proven and delivered awesome results since some strong dude in a cave invented weight training.

The compound moves include: squats, deadlifts, chin-ups, bent over row, upright row…and a few more. I cover all the top compound weight training exercises, muscle isolation exercises, and reveal my top training strategies in the book 'Strength Training Program 101: Build Muscle & Burn Fat…In Less Than 3 Hours Per Week'. It's available via Amazon and also features a bonus exercise demo guide to help readers master every move.

The reason compounds work so well is that they work various muscle groups at once and trigger the release of more anabolic hormones in the body. This basically means more muscle, less fat. We'll talk more about stimulating that anabolic response and the role of individual hormones in the body in the next chapter.

How Often - And How Long - Should You Be Training For?

How pissed off are you with your current body shape? How much do you want rid of the belly? How frustrating is it when you look in the mirror after weeks of training and dieting and see zero changes?

For many people the desperate need for change fires up their motivation levels to the extent where they're willing to train 5,6,7 days per week. They'll get up at stupid o'clock to do a fitness class before work. They'll drag themselves to the gym even when they're not feeling it after a long day.

Of course, that's the right attitude. You do have to work hard, do it consistently, and keep your nutrition on point to get the results you really want. But what if I told you that exercising barely three hours per week is enough to burn bodyfat, get lean and transform your bodyshape?

That's exactly what I'm telling you - if you train in the right manner. I'm sure you've already got the message that I'm not a fan of cardio. Weight training is the way because it does a 3 for 1 job: builds muscle, strips bodyfat and sculpts a leaner, more athletic physique overall. (There are countless other benefits as well such as improved heart health, stronger bones, better posture…these are all covered in my Strength Training Program 101 book).

Training in the right manner means lifting heavy weights with a lower amount of reps, and continually increasing the resistance on your muscles to trigger hypertrophy. The strain on your muscles will/should always leave you feeling sore as a result over the next 24-48 hours (sometimes longer for beginners), which means you must give your body sufficient rest to recover.

That's why I always recommend training **one day on, one day off** when it comes to lifting weights. (i.e. Monday, Wednesday, Friday). By focusing on various compound exercises you work many different muscle groups and ensure an all-over body workout more efficiently too - meaning your gym session can easily be finished in 45-60 mins. The only time I'm in the gym longer than an hour is if I'm wasting time talking to people or watching music videos of Rihanna on the TV. Or Beyonce. Or Taylor Swift.

Want a highly effective way to burn bodyfat - and keep it burning long after you step out of the gym? Then it's time to hit the weights section.

The Fat Loss Fast Lane

Did you ever watch the Olympics when you were a kid? Did it ever leave you a bit confused?

That's what happened with me. I loved the 100m sprint. It was fast, exciting and all of the guys competing were my vision of what a perfect athlete should look like. They always had strong powerful legs, broad shoulders, a rounded chest, bulging biceps, and perfect muscle definition - all with hardly a trace of bodyfat. To round it all off they were as quick as lightning.

Then I'd watch the 10,000m…and the runners were built like toothpicks. It looked likethey needed a meal more than any medal.

What was going on? Both groups of athletes were runners – but they had completely different physiques. I just couldn't get my head round it.

Turns out that these types of running trigger a different physiological response in the body. Long distance running is catabolic (aka breaks down muscle tissue) while sprinting is anabolic (builds muscle tissue).

The main reason for this is that the high intensity - all-out - power surge - of sprints in short bursts absolutely supercharges the body's production of growth hormone. One of the primary anabolic hormones, growth hormone is one of the key players in muscle growth and development.

Here's the big bonus: **<u>growth hormone also triggers lipolysis (fat breakdown) and also causes fatty acids to be utilised by the body</u>**. So it's essentially a two-for-one with sprint training - develop lean muscle while stripping fat at the same time.

Want to burn fat fast? Then it's time to start running fast. I mean flat out. Till you feel like your heart is going to burst through your chest.

On your marks. Get set…

Eight Reasons Why You Should Be Sprinting

Go out for a jog and you'll raise your heart rate, increase your metabolic rate, burns some calories, and then your body's systems will return back to normal fairly shortly afterwards.

Running at full speed - like you're being chased by an axe murderer - for just 10-15 seconds is on a whole other level. As I mentioned in the previous chapter, there's something special about sprinting that sparks a supercharged response in the endocrine system. It floods your body with muscle building, fat burning growth hormone, and sparks a surge of other anabolic hormones too.

Yet again, just like weight training, this means fat loss and muscle development at the same time. Now *that's* why Olympic sprinters - the men and the women - have bodies like Greek Gods. I don't think I've seen a female 100m sprint athlete without awesome abs.

Best of all: a single sprints training session can be done in as little as 15-20 mins. Below I list eight great reasons why you – and every fit and able person – should be sprinting.

#1 It can more than QUADRUPLE growth hormone production

Growth hormone is known for stimulating growth, cell regeneration and reproduction. As well as those fat burning benefits I've just described, growth hormone also plays various other roles in the body including enhancing immune system function.

So you can clearly see why doing anything that increases your levels of growth hormone is a good move when it comes to burning fat and improving your overall body shape.

Sprinting doesn't just give growth hormone a little boost – it supercharges it. A study published in The Journal of Sports Sciences in June 2002 showed that sprinting more than **quadrupled** growth hormone production.

Nine men completed two sprints – one for six seconds and another for 30 seconds – and had blood samples taken afterwards. Growth hormone levels were 450% higher after the 30 secs sprint compared to the short six second burst. These levels also stayed elevated for 90-120 minutes afterwards. Pretty amazing stuff!

#2 It kickstarts the other anabolic hormones too…

Sprinting may well turn you into an anabolic muscle growing, fat burning machine…because it also raises levels of the other primary anabolic hormones, testosterone and IGF1.

This was shown in another study published in The Journal of Strength And Conditioning Research in August 2011. The research involved 12 young men and highlighted that levels of testosterone and IGF1, along with growth hormone, were all elevated after various sprints involving distances of 100m-400m.

#3 It torches fat

Sprinting is like adding a heap of coal to your fat burning fire because it revs up your metabolism and keeps stripping fat long after your workout.

This form of training **<u>increased fat oxidation by 75%</u>**, according to research from February 2013. Researchers had 10 healthy men, aged 21-27, perform four 30 second bouts of cycle sprints, followed by almost five minutes of rest.

Aswell as the massive increase in fat oxidation, blood pressure levels were also shown to be reduced afterwards.

#4 It's a super efficient way to train

Your sprinting session should be finished in 15-20 mins. That's it. It simply involves intense bursts of speed over short distances, followed by quick breathers. Therefore it's a super efficient and ultra effective way to train.

Do it in the morning – on an empty stomach – for the best effect. In the previous study I mentioned above where the guys increased fat oxidation by 75%, they had all fasted overnight.

The significance of this is that your body's glycogen stores are lower after a period of fasting. If you haven't eaten since the previous evening when you sprint your body will turn to fatty acids for fuel…which equals an even better fat burn.

#5 It's a shortcut to a six-pack

The number one reason you've not got a six pack yet is not because you're not doing enough crunches. It's not because you had too much pasta on Tuesday night…

It's because your bodyfat levels are not low enough.

The abdominal muscles are there – but to get them on show you gotta remove the layer of fat that's camouflaging them. We've already seen how sprinting takes fat burning to new levels, while preserving and developing muscle mass. The exercise itself, thrusting your legs and arms forward powerfully at speed, also forces the abdominal muscles to work hard. I'd take 10 sprints over 1000 crunches any day.

#6 It improves heart health

Regular exercise is recommended for people with high blood pressure, and it appears that high intensity training is more effective than moderate exercise for improving the situation.

Comparing 30 minutes of moderate exercise to several bouts of high intensity (HIT) exercise, lasting 1-4 minutes, researchers concluded that HIT is "superior to CMT (continuous moderate training) for improving cardiorespiratory fitness".

Their findings published in the American Journal of Cardiovascular Disease in 2012 also showed that intense exercise was shown to have positive effects on arterial stiffness and insulin sensitivity.

#7 It strengthens the mind

Getting through a sprint session is tough, I won't lie. If it's your first time you'll feel like your heart is thumping, your mouth will be wide open trying to take in every tiny air particle, you'll think there's barely a drip of fuel left in the tank…

But that's the way it should be – and that's what will deliver all the other benefits ts listed above. Another big reason for sprinting is that it'll undoubtedly make you stronger mentally.

You've got to sprint so hard to the point where you think your body has nothing left to give. It's by pushing through and overcoming that mental battle that it'll strengthen your mind.

#8 It's a mood booster

We all know about the release of endorphins – feel good chemicals – that are stimulated by exercise, but this is heightened when you push yourself to the limit in this intense form of training. Especially when sprinting outside on a nice sunny morning.

My favourite time of year is spring and I love breathing in the fresh air with the sun shining on my sweaty face after an intense all-out sprint session. It sets you up for a positive day – I never have a bad day on a sprint day.

Different Types of Sprint Training

If you're still not convinced on sprinting then I'll eat my own stinking sweatyshoe after my sprint session tomorrow morning! Now we've discussed the main awesome benefits of sprint training, let's look at the three main options you have to get started.

- Standard sprints – on a flat surface, road or grass.
- Hill sprints – an incline will turn the intensity up a notch.
- Cycle sprints – all out pedalling with rest periods.

So let's just get this straight. Sprints supercharge growth hormone, get the body in an anabolic state to develop lean muscle mass, fire up fat burning, improve the health of your ticker, sculpt your six pack, strengthen the mind, make you feel amazing afterwards…and your workout is done in 15-20 minutes.

Have you pulled your running shoes on yet…?

Rapid Steps To Sprint Success

If you're ready to start sprinting then you had better get ready for some awesome results. But don't be thinking those results come easy. My friend introduced me to hill sprint training around 2011 – at a time when I thought I was in half decent shape and generally quite fit. An all-out sprint to the top of the hill, walk back down again, and repeat. What could be so hard about that?

The first sprint was pretty tough, I'd say 7/10. Reaching the top of the hill for my second one I was wheezing like an asthmatic, chest-infected chain-smoker. By the third I was gassed out – and thought I needed gas and air! That day I was planning on 10 hill sprints. I managed six.

The hill kicked my ass and showed me I wasn't nearly as fit as I thought I was. But...I was absolutely buzzing afterwards for still pushing through when I was really struggling after that third sprint.

I stuck at it, doing two sprint sessions per week outside on a hill near my house. My fitness improved quickly and I gradually increased the number of sprints and extended the distance as I progressed. Within a month the six pack abs I hadn't seen since I was about 18 were back. To be honest, my stomach was always flat and I could *feel* abdominal muscles – but up until that point you couldn't see them because they were well hidden by a layer of fat. Sprints stripped that fat away when all the other exercises I tried didn't.

You can benefit from the immense fat burn, while preserving and developing muscle as explained in the previous chapter. Here's how to get started and should progress as you gradually improve your sprinting performance and overall fitness.

ROOKIE (just starting out...)

Distance: 50-60 yards.

Sprints: 5-6.

>>> Head to your local park, or somewhere else outside, and locate a stretch of flat ground that's not very busy with people. (You want to be able to do your sprints uninterrupted without trying to swerve round people). >>> Choose a starting point and set a marker around 50-60 yards away, i.e. a park bench or street light. >>> Warm up for five minutes by jogging on the spot, doing star jumps, squats...and anything else that makes you feel slightly stupid outside! Seriously, the warm-up is important so also add-in various stretches for your legs and upper body too before you get started. >>> On your marks...sprint as fast as you possibly can to your marker point. As soon as you reach it walk back towards where you started, breathing in deep through your nose to get plenty of oxygen back in your lungs. >>> Once you get to the starting point, turn and set off again, running as fast as you can. >>> Repeat for 5-6 sprints.

INTERMEDIATE (have done sprints before, ready for more action...)

Distance: 100 yards.

Sprints: 8-9.

>>> Go to your local park, or somewhere else outside, and find a clear stretch of flat ground – or a spot with a slight incline. >>> Choose a starting spot and set a marker around 100 yards away. >>> Always make sure you warm up properly for five minutes before you begin. >>> Then, like above, sprint at maximum effort till you reach your marker and then walk back to the beginning. >>> Rinse and repeat for 8-9 sprints.

ADVANCED (Mr Bolt needs a 1 second head start on you...)

Distance: 120-150 yards.

Sprints: 10-12.

>>> Find a hill, or road with an incline (but not too steep...or else your calves will be on fire for the rest of the month). >>> Choose a starting point and set a marker further away this time, around 120-150 yards. >>> As ever, ensure you warm up well with stretches, jogging on the spot etc. >>> Using the same simple sprint/rest protocol, do this until you complete between 10 and 12 full sprints at maximum effort. Below I share with you my 11 point checklist to make sure you don't trip yourself up with schoolboy errors and instead get the most out of your sprint sessions.

Sprinter's Checklist

1. Set your alarm. Get up early to do your hill sprints before breakfast to maximise the fat burn.

2. Wear decent training shoes. Nice light ones.

3. Load music on to your iPhone...or whatever music player you use. You're gonna need good tunes to get you through to the end.

4. Wear tracksuit bottoms with a zip pocket...to keep your phone/music player in. I cracked the screen on my last iPhone after it fell out of my pocket when I was going at full-speed. It's also a pain in the ass running while holding your phone in your hand.

5. Take some handkerchiefs/toilet roll. Your nose will likely be dripping.

6. Don't forget to warm-up. Do a light jog and also take around 5 minutes doing some leg and arm stretches, running on the spot, bodyweight squats etc.

7. Take a bottle of water. You'll definitely be needing some h2o pronto afterwards.

8. Don't time yourself. It's a hassle and you're too busy fumbling around trying to start and stop the timer that you don't launch yourself off or finish properly. Just aim to go flat out from start to finish.

9. Set yourself a target number of sprints and stick to it. At least 5 as a rookie - and eventually work your way up to 12.

10. Don't give up. It's gonna be tough, no doubt about it but you gotta keep going.

11. Enjoy it. It may be tough physically and mentally just getting through the intense session but the buzz afterwards is amazing. The feel good endorphins will be bursting out your ears and it'll totally set you up for a great day.

Tabata Training

"Don't sit down, keep moving around…"

I can still hear the Australian voice repeating those words through the gym music system. I was a sweating, shaking, quivering mess and was wondering where the hell I was going to find the energy to get through the rest of the workout. I seriously thought I might spew - and that's exactly why there was always a sick bucket in the room during these intense sessions. My mate Alan Nisbet had plenty of fun filling that with his half-digested dinner on several occasions.

This was around 12 years ago and the first time I'd been introduced to 'Tabata' training…or done any proper high intensity interval training (HIIT) really. It was at the D-Unit Sports Combat Hub where I live in Alexandria, Scotland, and this special form of training was initially used to get the club's group of mixed martial arts stars in peak condition for their upcoming fights.

It involved doing various exercise drills at full capacity with very limited rest for almost an hour. It was punishing and, while I always thought I was fit as fuck, this proved I never really had the stamina I thought I had. The classes were then opened up to the local community and are still a big hit with hundreds of people every week at the D-Unit.

While I barely survived and just managed to hold in my puke, I loved how the Tabata system worked and was impressed after researching the science behind it. So much so that I now often apply it to the end of my weight training sessions, which I'll talk about later in this chapter.

Tabata training essentially involves 20 secs of exercise at maximum effort, followed by 10 secs rest, repeated for eight rounds. This short, sharp burst of training (just like sprints) is over very quickly…but the high level of intensity has the effect of elevating metabolism, and increasing the fat burn for up to 12 hours afterwards.

Now you're probably thinking, "I thought he said he didn't like cardio." I know, I'm a two-faced fucker. But I don't really class Tabata training or sprint training as cardio because they create such a unique physiological response in the body. Devised by Japanese scientist Dr Izumi Tabata, this professor did trials with Olympians and his findings were that Tabata training was more effective than other forms of HIIT for improving aerobic and anaerobic fitness.

Applying Tabata Training To Your Workouts

I like to throw in a Tabata style short session at the end of my weight training workouts to ramp up fat burning. This always involves lighter weights because you're pushing yourself harder for an extended period with minimal rest, rather than having a decent break in between three weightlifting sets.

For example, I might do squats with a 20kg weight bag resting on my shoulders, or bench press with a light weight. Twenty seconds work, 10 seconds rest, for the duration of the eight rounds.

I call it the workout 'finisher' and it definitely enhances the fat burning effect of your weights workout. There are plenty of free Tabata timer apps on the iTunes and Android stores that you can download to your phone for your workouts.

Personally, I'd recommend buying the 'Tabata Pro' timer app for £2.99. It's a cool, easy to use system, and also allows you to play your music at the same time (which can be a major help to get through a punishing Tabata round at the end of your workout).

Part Three

No Nonsense Nutrition

Sugar Ain't So Sweet

"Marc, what foods should I be cutting out to lose weight?"

"I don't really have a clue about a healthy diet. What should I be avoiding?"

"I've been eating low fat foods, but I've still not been losing any fat."

These are common questions I get from people via my weight training website, from friends, and even from my mum. But she still won't listen when I tell her to step away from the cakes. While intermittent fasting is always my number #1 piece of advice for anyone looking to burn bodyfat, making better food choices is obviously going to have a positive impact too. Stating the obvious with that one, but there's still a big misconception that eating high fat foods are what's making people fat.

Fat ain't the problem. <u>Sugar</u> is.

Consistently consume excessive amounts of sugar and it literally converts to bodyfat. Here's how it works…

Whenever we fill our bodies with too much fuel - which is very easy with high sugar foods - there's a glucose overload and the liver runs out of storage capacity. The excess sugar is converted into fatty acids and is then returned to the bloodstream. This is then stored as bodyfat in your belly, hips, chest and other areas you don't want it.

Too much sugar intake also results in insulin issues. Insulin is a key hormone in the body, and is released in high amounts whenever you eat or drink a "simple" carbohydrate, which includes the likes of white bread, white rice, baked white potato, bagels, croissants, cornflakes, cake, sugary drinks, beer, and anything that has high fructose corn syrup on the nutritional label.

When insulin levels are spiked the body's fat burning process is shut down so that the sugar that's just been consumed can be used for energy straight away. Sugar is shuttled into your muscles but, as soon as the muscle energy stores are full, the excess sugars are converted and stored as bodyfat.

So you can see that while it may taste oh so good at the time, sugar ain't so sweet for our bodyshape. It's also bad, very bad, for our health.

Cancer, heart disease, diabetes, metabolic syndrome and various other diseases have been strongly linked with over-consumption of refined sugar. Researchers at the University of California commented in the journal Nature that refined sugar contributes to around 35 million deaths around the world.

How Much Is Too Much?

The American Heart Association recommends that 37.5 grams (around 6 or 7 teaspoons) of added sugar is the daily limit for men, while 25g (around 5 teaspoons) is enough for women. To avoid going over the limit, ditching fizzy drinks and eating cakes and too much chocolate is wise move. And check the sugar content listed on nutritional labels on your food and drink.

Also, sugar is not always listed as sugar. Look out for the names of its man-made dodgy cousins including high fructose corn syrup, dried cane syrup and brown rice syrup. If there are several of them in the one food item then I'd steer clear.

Eating Clean Made Simple

Good nutrition accounts for about 70% of your fitness success, according to health experts.

Problem is, sticking to a healthy diet is where most of us struggle, right? If you're reading this now I'm guessing you've probably tried various diets or followed a nutrition plan devised by a PT in an attempt to get rid of excess bodyfat.

How did you find it? Was the food bland and boring? Was there too much meal prepping involved? Was it making you miserable trying to stick with it?

Fact is: if the 'diet' you're following is hard to maintain, not enjoyable, and feels like a strict military exercise then you're inevitably going to quit. That's the main reasons I take a different approach with personal training clients - and in my own life.

It's pointless me acting like a food Nazi, saying, "don't eat this…stay away from that…blah blah." Life's too short to put ourselves on ridiculous food bans. Everything in moderation is the way to go if it prevents us from quitting and eating a full tub of ice cream on a Wednesday night.

Four basic rules I stick by are:

- Eat clean Monday-Friday…and live a little at the weekend.

- Include plenty of whole foods in your diet (the stuff that grows in the ground and on trees).

- Cook fresh as much as possible.

- Limit sugar and processed foods (i.e. ready meals, sweets etc).

Enjoy your usual Chinese takeaway meal - but save it for the weekend. Have a little chocolate - just make sure it's not a king size bar. You get the idea.

If you follow those four basic rules, and combine them with intermittent fasting and regular exercise, you can't go wrong. You'll still be burning fat while not subjecting yourself to an extreme diet or unhealthy ways of eating that will only result in failure eventually.

My book 'Strength Training Nutrition 101: Build Muscle & Burn Fat Easily…A Healthy Way Of Eating You Can Actually Maintain' goes into much more detail on this. It also lists my top food sources for protein, carbohydrates and fat, guidelines on how much of these macronutrients you should be taking in based on your body type, and more.

While my approach is not to be the food police, I've still pulled together a list of foods that it's advisable to **avoid** as much as possible if you want to successfully burn fat and get leaner.

#1 Fizzy drinks

Cola, Pepsi, 7-Up…all these sugar-laden fizzy drinks are bad news for your waistline and your health. I already covered the dangers of too much sugar in the last chapter and how it converts to fat in the body. Downing fizzy drinks is like shuttling spoonful after spoonful of sugar into your mouth. Swap it for water, or diluting juice.

#2 White bread

White bread is not good for you. It lacks the fibre and several other nutrients that whole grain bread provides. Adding to the problem is the fact that white bread is not naturally white - the flour is chemically bleached to give it that colour. Yep, bleached. Best giving that a miss too.

#3 Cakes, sweets

I'm not sure I have to explain why here, but I will anyway. Cakes and sweets contain large amounts of sugar, often with hydrogenated fats which are damaging to your health. Remember, what I said about eating clean Monday-Friday and relaxing your diet a little at the weekend? Cakes and sweets should be left till the weekend.

#4 Beer/lager

Beer and lager will hamper your fat burning attempts for various reasons. Firstly, they contain more calories than most other alcoholic drinks. There are usually at least 200 calories in a pint of beer and I know guys who can easily drink 8-10 pints a night at the pub.

When we're heading home drunk we usually grab some sort of takeaway food, don't we? That's causing another problem because alcohol affects the body's ability to metabolise calories, causing them to be stored as fat rather than glycogen. When we're hungover the next day there's nothing healthy on the menu, only junk food will do! All in all, beer and lager are best avoided if you want to successfully burn fat.

#5 Margarine

My mum put margarine on my sandwiches all through primary school - it's no wonder I've turned out like this! Seriously, I don't know why this stuff even continues to sell. Margarine surged in popularity a couple of decades ago as an alternative to butter because there was the misconception that saturated fat was bad for us. Turns out it's the other way round. Margarine contains man-made trans-fats which are denatured and unhealthy to the body. Butter is the healthier, more natural and tastier choice.

#6 Vegetable oils

This follows the same kind of argument as above. Vegetable oils grew in popularity when health experts demonised saturated fats, believing they were bad for our health and caused heart disease. It is now widely accepted that saturated fat plays various important roles in the body including the manufacture of hormones and immune function. Vegetable oils meanwhile, such as sunflower, corn and canola oil, are less than healthy and are hard for the body to break down when heated.

Why Energy Drinks Are To Be Avoided

Every time I walk into the gym I can expect to count at least two or three drinks cans sitting in a corner on the floor.

There are countless brands of energy drinks being sold these days and there's a misconception that these will help you achieve your health and fitness goals quicker. I often see people downing them to get through their workouts, clearly thinking it'll give them a boost in performance and fire them up for a better workout. And a better workout equals more fat burnt, right?

In the case of energy drinks, no. In fact, it's completely defeating the purpose. You might feel wired and charged up due to the sky high levels of caffeine in these energy drinks, but some of them also contain up to **17 teaspoons of sugar!** This is more than DOUBLE the recommended amount of daily added sugar. As explained earlier, excess sugar is eventually stored as bodyfat. So for anyone looking to burn fat and lose weight, drinking a sugar-laden energy drink to try and achieve this is a pretty stupid move.

Along with bags of caffeine, these drinks also contain all sorts of other unnatural ingredients you've probably never heard of before. I bought three cans of big name brand energy drinks to draw a comparison and I was shocked by the huge number of flavourings, colourings, and other questionable additives in them. Sure, there were some vitamins and natural ingredients included, but these are negligible in my opinion, given that excess sugar robs the body of vitamins and minerals anyway.

Here's how those drinks stacked up:

Brand A

Sugar - 55g (13 teaspoons) per 500ml can.

Ingredients - 20.

Brand B

Sugar - 69g (17 teaspoons) per 500ml can.

Ingredients - 14.

Brand C

Sugar - 39g (9 teaspoons) per 355ml can.

Ingredients - 15.

These cans went straight into the bin after I checked them out and made the comparison for the purposes of this chapter. Below are five strong reasons I'd recommend you do the same.

5 Reasons For Ditching Energy Drinks

#1 The caffeine content can be dangerously high

Caffeine increases alertness and provides a boost in energy but too high doses – while mixed with other ingredients and/or alcohol – can potentially be lethal. Several deaths around the world have been linked to various energy drinks. I won't single out any particular brands because lawsuits are still ongoing in some cases, but if you've been consuming energy drinks it's worth doing some research online before you gulp another drop. You might be shocked at what you discover.

#2 Way too much sugar

One word for the amount of added sugar in the energy drinks cans I've mentioned - ridiculous! Just imagine dropping 17 teaspoons of sugar into a pint glass of water and then drinking it. That's basically what people are doing when they consume this stuff.

Refined sugar in all its man-made forms (including the likes of 'high fructose corn syrup', 'sucrose', 'glucose syrup' etc) is the enemy to good health. Over consumption of sugar is strongly linked to all the big major diseases including cancer, heart disease and diabetes.

#3 They are NOT the same as sports drinks designed for performance enhancement

Sports drinks contain water, smaller amounts of sugar and minerals such as potassium and sodium that are lost during intense physical activity. Many top brands are used to good effect by athletes as they enhance hydration and provide carbohydrates for energy - but don't have the same massive amounts of sugar or stimulating effects as high caffeine energy drinks.

#4 There could be long-term effects medical experts are not aware of yet

The energy drinks market has exploded in recent years and there's little research available on the long term effects of consuming these products regularly.

On the websitesharecare.com, Dr Michael Breus PhD warns that we're still in the early stages of learning about "the full range of effects of energy drinks on physical and mental health, as well as sleep."

#5 There are safer, healthier alternatives

There are a variety of natural foods, drinks and supplements that you can take that can give you an energy boost pre-workout. One unexpected source of energy that is growing in popularity among athletes, particularly endurance runners, is beetroot juice.

It's believed that beetroot juice increases blood and oxygen flow in the body. That's undoubtedly why athletes were using it at the London 2012 Olympics and why US marathon runner Ryan Hall always downs a glass to improve his run time.

I gave it a try last month...and it was too gaggingly disgusting to try again. I share an easier, tastier, simpler pre-workout drink option with you in Part Four which is like rocket fuel for your exercise sessions.

Keeping Your Calories In Check

Calories are important when it comes to fat loss, but do you really want to count how many are in your meals every day? No, me neither.

Life's too short to be doing sums in your head every time you take a bite to eat or have a drink. Fortunately, you don't have to because there's an awesome app worth using to help you keep your calories in check and to optimise your daily nutrition.

I'll come to that soon, but first let's talk about calories and their effect on your weight levels. A calorie, also known as a kilocalorie, is the measure of energy within the food and drink we consume. It provides us with fuel for our daily activities…including those tough weights and sprint sessions I was talking about earlier.

If we regularly take in more calories than we use up every day then naturally we'll gain weight. The reverse is true: to lose weight we must be in a caloric deficit. How many calories we burn each day depends on various factors including age, genetics, sex, and how active you are. A postman out and about delivering mail for hours each day is going to burn more calories than an office worker sitting at their desk all day.

For me personally, I naturally have a high metabolism and exercise 3-4 days per week, meaning that I must take in more calories particularly on workout days to ensure I don't lose weight.

If you're overweight and want to shed bodyfat, it's a must that you cut back on calories until you hit your target. Then you can make adjustments once you've achieved your aim.

There are a couple of ways to figure how many calories an active person generally needs each day. The first is this simple equation which provides an approximate number:

* Weight loss: bodyweight in pounds x 12 = number of daily calories.

* Weight maintenance: bodyweight in pounds x 15 = number of daily calories.

* Weight gain: bodyweight in pounds x 18 = number of daily calories.

This is a formula that gives you a very rough idea, but our bodies are all different and remember there are various other factors which contribute to your caloric needs.

That's where the MyFitnessPal app comes in. It's an amazing tool for not only figuring out an accurate picture of your calorie requirements based on your specific fitness goals, it also helps you keep on top of your nutrition overall easily.

Rather than counting calories, grams of protein, carbs or how much fat is in your foods, you can simply scan barcodes on packaging with the MyFitnessPal app or type in the name of foods and it automatically works it all out for you. Your nutritional stats are easily saved into a daily food diary and you can take full charge of your nutrition in just a few minutes per day.

I use this app with online personal training clients, as do many other health and fitness professionals around the world. While it's not a necessity for you to track your calories or use a food diary in the long term, it's a key tool to use until you burn fat and lose enough weight to hit your fitness target.

If you're looking to burn fat fast and have struggled to lose weight for a while, a perfect combination would be:

intermittent fasting + weight training three days per week + a daily caloric deficit. Throw a single 15 minute sprints session per week into the mix and you'll inevitably smash your goal.

To use the MyFitnessPal app you'll have to set up a free account. After that it's fairly easy to use but there are several features you might want to explore, such as saving meal recipes. You can learn how to use the app properly via this YouTube demo video:
https://www.youtube.com/watch?v=fu9RKqlmD1Q&t=179s

Delay Your Post-Workout Shake

Have you been told to guzzle a protein shake straight after your workout for maximum muscle, minimal fat?

It's common sense advice. Gulp down a shake filled with the right amount of protein and carbs to flood your system with nutrients. Then the body can get to work on developing muscle and sculpting that awesome new physique you're aiming for.

I did that for the best part of 10 years. Dropping the dumbbell for the last rep of my workout in the gym, grabbing my shaker (already with protein powder inside), and running to fill it up with water so I could have my shake immediately.

The body is in a catabolic (muscle tissue breakdown) state after an intense workout and that flips to anabolic (muscle building) when you provide it with the right nutrients for repair and development.

My thinking process was: the sooner that healthy protein shake hits my stomach the better my body transformation will be. After busting my balls in a heavy weights session, I want to make sure I capitalise on all my hard work.

A while ago that approach has changed - slightly - thanks to the wisdom of the sports nutrition mastermind Ori Hofmekler. (I referred to Ori's work in Part One). In a fascinating interview with American fitness guru Dr Chad Waterbury, Ori Hofmekler revealed that delaying your post-workout shake/meal by 30-60 mins after your training session you can maximise fat burning.

Ori said: "Exercise only initiates the first phase of fat breakdown; it does not grant the completion of the fat-burning process. After exercise there's a substantial increase in the level of circulating free fatty acids coming from adipose tissue, and unless these are mobilized to the liver and muscle for final utilization, most of them will be re-esterfied into triglycerides and re-deposited back in the fat tissues.

"Yes, all your hard work to burn fat will be wasted! In order to grant an effective completion of the fat-burning process you must manipulate your muscle to suck in the circulating free fatty acids that were released by exercise.

"And the way to do that is to wait for 30-60 minutes after exercise before having your recovery meal."

There you have it - exercise is only half of the fat burning process. By delaying your post-workout shake/meal by 30 minutes to one hour this prevents fatty acids from being drawn back into fat tissues; thereby maximising your fat loss efforts.

The interview with Ori, titled 'The Truth About Post Workout Nutrition', is a detailed and very interesting read. Well worth checking out and you can do so by visiting:http://chadwaterbury.com/the-truth-about-post-workout-nutrition/

One Positive Habit Per Week

Meet Steven. A 30-year-old construction worker who has just started dating a girl for the first time since has last relationship ended four years ago.

He's been piling on the pounds for years, not really bothering much about it, but suddenly decides now is the time to sort out his health and fitness (again). He wants to improve his appearance, be more confident…thinking it'll help him hang onto his new girlfriend.

Steven's biggest issue - his diet. He boozes every Friday and Saturday (sometimes the odd weeknight too), he rarely sleeps well as a result, he eats takeaways 3-4 days per week, dinner is usually followed by 4 or 5 biscuits, he drinks a two litre bottle of Coke while at work, and the only time he sees vegetables are when he walks past them in the supermarket while heading straight for the pizzas.

Not exactly the healthiest of lifestyles and Steven knows it. There's plenty to change and he's determined to do it because he wants to drop two stones, maybe even three if possible.

So, the diet begins. No to booze, no to biscuits, no to pizza, no to the takeaway meals. He's gone cold turkey on the junk. And it's yes to low fat yoghurts, tasteless 'healthy' microwave meals, and generally starving himself to try and get rid of the flab.

Fast forward three weeks: he's lost barely 3lbs, is miserable, been arguing with his girlfriend as a result…and is so pissed off with it all that he's just ordered a large Big Mac Meal, two double cheeseburgers, a strawberry milkshake, and a donut at McDonald's.

True story. Although his name's not actually Steven - and I think he ordered 10 chicken nuggets and an apple pie aswell. Here's the moral of the story: if you try to change everything at once it'll likely end up in failure.

There's quite a lot to take in from this book, training and nutrition wise, especially if you've not done much exercise until now or didn't really have a clue about following a healthy diet.

This can mean an entire lifestyle change and wrestling with a lot of bad old habits. These are like programmes we've created over years…and it's not a straightforward 'deprogramming' process simply because you've read this book.

I'll put it this way: if you try to implement everything at once you'll likely fuck things up. And I don't want you to fuck things up.

These exercise and nutritional strategies already covered in this book have long been proven for blitzing bodyfat and helping people get in much better shape. But it's wise to introduce these positive changes - and remove the negative ones - *gradually* in order for you to be successful.

Otherwise you'll likely end up feeling overwhelmed and it'll create resistance within you to keep pushing on. So what should you do?

When it comes to exercise focus on one thing at a time - and then build upon it.

When it comes to your nutrition make one change at a time - and then build upon this too.

When I take on new personal training clients, I ask them to fill in a short questionnaire about their diet and nutrition so I can get a clear picture of their eating habits and to see what we can improve.

In most cases, there are numerous foods and drinks they should be cutting back on in order to see the changes they want. There are often many healthy foods they should be including more of.

They're desperate to hear about all of these to help them hit their health and fitness goals sooner. But it won't do any good bombarding them with everything at once. It leads to information overload, trying to make too many changes at once, and effectively moving onto to a restrictive 'diet'. I don't do diets. Instead, we make gradual changes by introducing **one positive habit per week**.

Where should you start? What should be implemented in what order? I think it's important to put core practices in place first; the ones that will get quickest results. Then you can keep adding in one new positive habit per week.

For example, if you currently go out jogging twice per week to try and burn fat then I'd swap that for three weight training sessions at the gym. This is a core foundational change to your exercise regime.

The following week you could focus on your diet and get started with intermittent fasting. Again, this is probably the best place to start when it comes to diet and nutrition. Stay focused only on skipping breakfast for that week, with no other diet distractions.

By week two, you've proven you can stick with intermittent fasting and now it's time to build upon that. You realise your high sugar intake is one of the main reasons for being overweight, so you resolve to only have dessert after your dinner one day this week instead of 5-6 days per week. This is your target for week two, don't worry about fixing anything else in your diet for now.

By week three you're not only gaining momentum, but you're gaining confidence and strengthening your willpower because you've achieved your goals so far. This week's positive habit to add to the previous two - cook double the amount of food for dinner this week and take the other serving into work the next day. Your freshly cooked food is a much better option to the junk food you've been buying in the work canteen or from the fast food joint down the road.

You see where I'm going with this? It's easy to understand, easy to implement and, most importantly, it's much easier to maintain. Don't worry, if you have the odd slip-up. We all do, and again it's because we're so used to our old negative habits even if they're not good for our health.

The key is to stay focused on one positive habit per week and do your best to achieve it each day. Keep stacking those habits, keep building your confidence, and watch as your burn fat faster than you've ever done before.

Part Four:

Fat Burning Hacks

Training In The Morning On An Empty Stomach

Remember being told that breakfast is the "most important meal of the day"?

Maybe for kids going to school to help them focus on their education without their bellies grumbling. For adults? The health benefits of skipping breakfast extend way beyond burning fat and staying lean, but actually include improved digestion, detoxification, cell regeneration, the list goes on.

After doing plenty of research into why intermittent fasting was good for me, I was more than content to give brekkie a break. But no food in my stomach before my workouts? **I'm not advising this for lifting heavy weights**, but when it comes to an early morning sprints session an empty belly is the only way to go.

It was only after I began early morning sprint training sessions with my mate Ryan that I began experimenting with exercising on an empty stomach. We got up at 7am to get ready for sprints and I quickly wolfed down a bowl of porridge, thinking I'd really need those carbs to get me through the tough high intensity session. Ryan, as usual, decided to have his breakfast later in the morning and did his sprints on an empty stomach.

Here's what happened: by the third sprint I was close to spewing, the food felt like a heavy weight in my stomach, and I developed an instant headache. Next time around, I sprinted on an empty stomach and, despite worrying I'd be dizzy because there was no food fuel in my body, I performed much better.

Guess what else I noticed a few weeks down the line? The thin layer of flab around my belly had disappeared and my abs were properly on show again. As described earlier, sprint training has a huge fat burning effect, but combining this with training in the morning on an empty stomach moved things up a gear.

American doctor and health guru, Joseph Mercola, is a big proponent of exercising early in the morning on an empty stomach. For people aiming to burn fat, he says that working out in the AM while still in a fasted state following sleeping is a wise move.

He explains that the combination of fasting and exercising maximises the impact of cellular factors and catalysts, which result in the breakdown of fat for energy. Training on an empty stomach effectively forces your body to burn up fat.

Here's another reason to drag yourself out of bed and exercise in the AM…you're much more likely to stick to your weekly training regime. When you training in the morning you can't make the excuse that you ran out of time, or that a meeting came up, or that you had to work late at the office. If training is your start to the day, then it's less likely to be ditched for something else.

An Energy Booster

When I say training on an empty stomach, I'm not being *completely* honest. I've usually given myself a cheeky wee boost. It's something you might drink every day, something you might love the smell of, and something that'll not only supercharge your training but boost fat burning by around 10%.

Your cup is served in the next chapter.

Supercharge Your Workouts With Black Coffee

If you're worried that you'll struggle to get through a tough workout in the morning on an empty stomach, then relax and pour yourself a cuppa.

A black coffee will give your bags of beans in the gym. The caffeine will flow through your system and provide more energy than any bowl of cereal. Best of all: it's been proven to take stoke your fat burning fire.

The caffeine in coffee not only provides the fuel you need for training, but it can cause fatty acids to be used for energy rather than glycogen. Studies have shown that coffee also speeds up metabolism and fat oxidation, which means more fat is burned throughout the day.

I'm guessing there are one of two thoughts going through your mind right now…

"Can it *really* be that effective at burning fat?" or "…I fucking HATE coffee!"

I've lost count of the amount of people who've told me they can't drink the stuff. That it makes them feel sick. That they'd rather drink a shot of their own piss. (Well, maybe not the last statement).

I'll be honest, I was never really a big fan of coffee. In fact, I'm still not…but I neck a cup of it anyway because of the awesome effect it has on my training. One cup of black coffee (yes, no sugar or cream) and made from ground coffee beans rather than instant granules that have been ridiculously processed and robbed the coffee of its natural antioxidants.

Yes, coffee actually contains antioxidants that can clear out toxins in the body, supposedly slow ageing, and apparently reduce the risk of cancer. To enjoy these benefits make your coffee using organic beans or freshly ground coffee, rather than the instant garbage. And go easy on it as health experts recommend no more than 400mg of caffeine (roughly three mugs of coffee) per day.

7 Reasons Why Having A Black Coffee Pre-Workout Is A Hot Idea

1. Performance boost

Coffee can be the difference between shaving a few seconds off your running time or adding a couple more exercises to your training regime.

This was proven back in 1992 when a group of athletes were given 3g of coffee before a 1500m treadmill run. The study, published in the British Journal of Sports Medicine showed that those who drank the coffee finished their run 4.2 secs faster on average than the control group.

2. Increased energy

The caffeine in coffee can provide a much-needed charge to your batteries before exercise. Just don't go nuts as excessive caffeine intake has been shown to have side effects such as increased heart rate and insomnia.

Remember, medics widely recommend that no more than 400mg of caffeine (three mugs) is consumed per day, while the limit is 200mg for pregnant women.

3. More fat is burned

Some health experts say that coffee can increase your basal metabolic rate by around 10%, while others say as much as 20%. I expect the figure varies from person to person, but what's not in question is that coffee can speed up your metabolism.

This means more calories burned and more fat melted away.

4. Improved focus

Along with more energy to burn during exercise, black coffee also keeps you alert and provides an increase in mental focus. This helps you stick with it and get the most out of each workout.

5. Can help the unfit become more active

A group of sedentary men hopped on exercise bikes after drinking caffeine for a study in 2012. Researchers were so impressed by the performance of these unfit guys that they reckon the boost given by caffeine could "motivate sedentary men to participate in exercise more often and so reduce adverse effects of inactivity on health."

6. Reduced muscle soreness

Drinking coffee before exercise can reduce muscle soreness post-workout by up to 48%, according to the following study published in the March 2007 issue of Journal Of Pain.

7. It's a healthy alternative to energy drinks

The popularity of energy drinks has exploded to the point that it is now a multi-billion dollar industry. As mentioned earlier, health experts have repeatedly warned about the dangers of these drinks due to the mixture of high levels of caffeine, sugar and various other ingredients.

Best steering clear when there's a healthier, safer alternative. Now you have seven good reasons to drink coffee. Serve up one mug – without the cream and sugar – 30-60 mins before you next exercise to stir up those energy levels.

Give Green Tea The Green Light

Are you a tea with two sugars and milk kinda person? Do you have 3,4,5 cups per day…maybe 17 when you're hungover or feeling like shit?

Why not ditch at least some of those cups for **green tea** instead to give your body a fat-burning boost? I'm drinking my second cup of the day (in my special Kylie Minogue mug) as I type this.

If you want to give your body a helping hand to slim down the waistline and lose any jiggly bits, then it's time to give green tea the green light. Scientific studies have shown that there's something quite special going on with those green tea leaves and its fat burning magic is becoming well known.

Green contains catechins which naturally raise levels of the key fat burning hormone norepinephrine. Norepinephrine elevates metabolism levels and increases the rate of fatty acid utilisation…meaning that your cuppa green can turn you into a blubber burning boss!

What Brand And How Many Cups?

This is where you'll have to do a bit of research because the quality of tea leaves and catechin content can vary dramatically. This is all down to where the tea plant is grown, if it's classed as organic or not, and how it's actually processed. Studies have shown that even the brew time and water temperature can affect the amount of catechins in the cuppa.

If you're looking for a top quality brew than Green Tea Lovers (greentealovers.com) is a good place to start. The New York based company sources high quality, organic, Fair Trade green tea from around the world and boasts that its teas have "ultra high antioxidant levels". Otherwise, if you choose to buy at your local supermarket then it's worth paying a little more for a better quality brand, looking out for organic tea bags.

Green tea reaches its fat-burning potential with around 400-500 milligrams of ECGC—the most active catechin—per day. That's around four cups of strongly brewed tea.

A simple alternative is to opt for a green tea extract (GTE) supplement. GTE pills are becoming more widely used by people looking to cut their bodyfat levels. They are sold cheaply on leading sports supplements websites such as MyProtein.com and allow you to take green tea in a more concentrated form and fully benefit from the fat burning effects of green tea. These tablets are natural, safe, and effective for weight loss, backed up by many customer reviews online.

Remember to check the labels and not to exceed the recommended dosage because GTE also contains caffeine.

The Magic Of Lemon Water

This last chapter will finish oh so beautifully with one of the first things I do every morning. I repeated it and repeated it constantly until it became a habit just like brushing my teeth. Now it's second nature and undoubtedly one of the best things I do for my health.

One pint glass.

Filled with lukewarm water.

And the juice of half a lemon.

So easy to do. Also so easy not to do when you're scrambling around late for work or getting the kids ready for school. But if you make a conscious effort to have this refreshing drink for at least a month you'll discover it's an amazing start to each day. It can also boost your fat-burning efforts because lemon juice contains pectin fibre which helps reduce your appetite.

There are plenty other health benefits you can experience simply by buying in 3 or 4 lemons per week and adding the juice to water every morning. One of the first, and most obvious, reasons for doing this is that we're typically most dehydrated when we first wake up. The combination of taking in no fluids while we're snoozing, combined with sweating during our sleep, results in dehydration.

Of course, the tell-tale sign that you need some h2o in your system is if your pee is coloured and not clear. This is usually the situation in the morning. This is your cue to head to kitchen, heat a pint of water a little, pour into a pint glass, and then squeeze the juice of half a lemon before drinking.

Not only does it taste awesome, there are many reasons for enjoying a glass of lemon water. Below are just some of the main ones.

8 Benefits Of Drinking Lemon Water

#1 Better digestion

Lemon juice has antibacterial qualities and helps rid the intestines of toxins. Too much processed food in the typical Western diet often leads to digestive issues, such as constipation and heartburn for many people. These are clear signs that your body's struggling to break down what you've been consuming and this can lead to toxins floating around in your system.

The antibacterial effect of lemon juice helps flush toxins and bacteria, which is important at the start of your day before you continue eating more food.

#2 Immune system boost

Lemons and other citrus fruits contain high amounts of vitamin C, which is one of the most important antioxidant vitamins for boosting the immune system. Vitamin C helps protect cells from damaging free radicals, is needed for healing wounds, and contributes to maintaining strong bones and teeth.

#3 It contains other vitamins and minerals

While not on the same scale as vitamin C, lemon juice also contains the B vitamins riboflavin, folate, thiamin and B6. These are important for metabolism, helping the body convert carbohydrates, proteins and fats into glucose to be used for energy. A deficiency in B vitamins leads to tiredness and fatigue.

Lemon juice also contains the minerals magnesium, calcium and is particularly high in potassium, which is good for heart health and the function of your brain and nervous system.

#4 Cancer protection

Compounds called limonoids are found in lemons. These also have antioxidant properties, helping to destroy free radicals in the body. Limonoids also have the ability to help prevent the development and growth of cancer cells, according to a report in the April 2005 issue of the Journal of Nutrition. Tested against human cancer cells, limonoids not only halted their growth but were also responsible for the death of the cancer cells.

#5 Clearer skin

The antioxidants in lemon juice help to decrease blemishes on your skin. As it's detoxifying to your blood, it helps maintain a healthy complexion.

#6 Blood sugar regulation

Another compound found in lemons called hesperidin can have a positive impact on the function of enzymes in the body that affect blood sugar levels. As this can help lower blood sugar levels, the result is that this compound can protect the body from the development of diabetes. This was concluded in the January 2010 issue of the Journal of Clinical Biochemistry and Nutrition, which also reported that hesperidin has cholesterol-lowering effects too.

#7 Helps prevent kidney stones

Kidney stones are solid mineral formations that can build up in the kidneys. The citric acid found in lemons is just what the doctor ordered for preventing kidney stones. Health experts report that more citrate in your system can halt the formation of calcium stones. Lemons and limes have the most citric acid, while oranges, grapefruits and berries also contain large amounts.

#8 Helps fight viral infections

Again this is down to the antibacterial qualities of lemons. In studies it has been shown to kill deadly diseases such as malaria, cholera, diptheria, and typhoid. Squeeze the life out of pathogens with some fresh lemon water.

Want to kickstart a leaner, healthier lifestyle and do what you can to protect yourself from various illnesses? A simple pint of lemon water every day could go a long way to helping you achieve this.

Conclusion

In four parts, 21 chapters, and nearly 17,000 words we've gone over a wide variety of *physical* actions you can take to Burn Fat Fast.

Changes to your meal timing, what's included in your meals, and what you should avoid like the plague. We've looked at your weekly training regime, why weight training is much more effective at burning fat than cardio and why intense sprint training is the secret to a leaner, stronger body.

You can now make some tweaks that'll contribute to your body sculpting mission such as delaying your post-workout meal and building upon one positive habit per week.

You're now armed to go to war on your bodyfat with fat burning hacks that are not only easy to implement, but have been proven to deliver results time and again.

I've saved the biggest hack of all until now…

One that is the superglue for holding everything else together and making sure it doesn't break.

I'm talking about hacking your **mindset** and forcing a complete shift from your usual pattern of thinking when it comes to your health and fitness - and your self image.

All of the strategies I've described up until now work well for burning fat, improving your fitness levels and getting in great shape. I have zero doubt that if you implement these exercise and dietary principles as described that you'll achieve your particular goal; whether that's getting rid of some stubborn belly fat or losing a considerable amount of weight.

Forget how many times you may have failed in the past, this is a new start and you now have highly effective strategies that have spawned countless success stories. Best of all: the approach in this book doesn't involve any crazy yo-yo dieting or extreme exercise routine you cannot maintain.

It's do-able, manageable, and sustainable in the long term. You can achieve great results - but I want you to **maintain them**. That's why we must conclude by focusing on mindset right now.

This was the big issue for a recent personal training client of mine called Johnny. He'd been working with another PT for months, wasn't happy with his rate of progress, and decided to quit.

A couple of months later, pissed off with the weight piling on and with another gust of willpower, he asked to join my 10 week training and nutrition coaching programme. He was two stones overweight but after looking closely at his diet, it wasn't exactly the worst.

We changed up his gym routine to focus on heavy weight training with compound exercises and he was already damn good at many of these moves. In fact, he was a boss at squats and deadlifts and was soon lifting more than me.

After a couple of weeks it became apparent what was really holding Johnny back…his mindset and doubts about what he was capable of.

He told me: "When I tried to lose weight the last time around I got rid of just a few pounds but that was it. Every time I stepped on the scales I knew it would be the same. I kept thinking, 'is this a waste of time?', 'am I doing the exercises wrong?'

"I stepped up my training to six days per week and then ended up even more pissed off because I wasn't getting the results for the amount of effort I was putting in.

"I'm always willing to work hard but it always seems like I'm so far away from getting anywhere."

The more he spoke the clearer our #1 problem became: Johnny was already defeated before he began.

Have you ever stopped to properly listen to your thoughts as you work your ass off to become healthier and fitter? That nagging, annoying, relentless inner critic whispering words of doubt in your head, even when you're clearly working hard towards your goal.

"I still can't see any changes in my body, feels like I'm getting nowhere…"

"Maybe I'm just not working hard enough, maybe I'm just doing it all wrong…"

"Am I wasting my time at the gym?"

"My diet hasn't been great the past couple of days, who am I kidding I can lose this weight?"

Who needs enemies when you've got the harshest critic around inside your own head? I don't care who you are or what weight, age, or nationality you are, we all have insecurities and body image issues to some degree. But there are two very important steps you must take to develop the right mindset for achieving your goals.

#1 Stand guard over your mind.

Don't let your inner critic take over. He'll take full charge and fuck everything up. When those doubts, negative thoughts and criticisms start creeping in, bat them right out of the park.

This may take a firm conscious effort for a while because many of us have become masters at beating ourselves up. Instead, keep praising yourself for the positive action steps you're taking every day to become a healthier, stronger, better version of yourself.

#2 Act like you've <u>already achieved</u> what you're aiming for.

If you're always thinking in terms of "I want this…" or "I want to achieve that…", you're creating a sense of lack. You're simply reinforcing that you're not where you want to be, and it's going to make it all the harder to get there. Instead, behave like you're ***already*** lean, strong and in the best shape of your life.

The subconscious mind can't tell a white lie from what's real. Keep feeding it this image of you having already achieved your health and fitness goals - while you continue to work hard - and the body will eventually follow suit.

I said at the beginning of this book that burning fat is easy…and I'm sticking to my guns. Intermittent fasting is easy…much easier than trying out 23,056 different diets in your lifetime.

Limiting your sugar intake every day is easy…much easier than developing diabetes, heart disease or some other serious illness.

Keeping an eye on your calories is easy…introducing one positive habit per week is easy…as is ditching energy drinks, downing a pint of lemon water in the morning, and giving green tea a try.

What's not quite so easy is sprint training. In fact, the first time you do it you may even feel like your heart's going to burst through your chest. But it's so ridiculously effective for burning bodyfat that you'd be a fool to not give it a go. One 15 minute session per week is all it takes and, while it's tough as hell, real change only occurs outside of your comfort zone.

As for weight training, I've long argued that this is the most effective form of exercise for men and women looking to develop a strong, lean, toned body. I touched upon the importance of compound exercises, lifting heavy, and why lifting weights just three days per week is all that's required to get in great shape.

I go into much more detail on this in my book 'Strength Training Program 101: Build Muscle & Burn Fat…In Less Than 3 Hours Per Week'. However, you can also download my exercise guide e-book for free by visiting: www.weighttrainingistheway.com/exercise-demos

I hope you've enjoyed reading this book and, if so, I'd be hugely grateful if you left a review on Amazon.

You now have the knowledge and tools to Burn Fat Fast, and transform your overall bodyshape and health.

Work hard. Have faith. Believe in yourself.

Strength Training Program 101: Build Muscle & Burn Fat

In Less Than 3 Hours Per Week

By

Marc McLean

Introduction

Strength Training Is THE Way to a better body, optimal health and improved fitness.

This book promises the way to more muscle and less fat – and the strategies included here deliver. But there's so much more to gain from going down the path laid out in these pages.

Looking great. Feeling amazing. Increased confidence. Achieving what you thought you never could have before in the gym – and seeing that success have a positive knock-on effect in other areas of your life.

That's the ultimate aim of *Strength Training Program 101* - to help you <u>become a stronger, healthier, better version of you</u>.

Lifting weights (heavy please), strengthening and sculpting your body goes way beyond the physical. It has an incredible impact on your mental health and wellbeing, and your whole outlook and approach to life.

May sound a bit over the top, but I've experienced it personally and witnessed it with plenty of clients and friends time and again over the years.

The discipline, dedication and personal enjoyment you gain from all your achievements in the gym can help change your entire vibe! Don't be surprised if you then start seeing unexpected changes in relationships, career, or other areas of your life.

I've been lifting weights since I was a seriously skinny 16-year-old and made countless mistakes along the way. There's no need for you to make the same errors because I've crammed in

18 years' worth of knowledge and experience into these 110 pages.

Building a Strong, Athletic, Lean Physique…

Let's be clear straight away: this book is all about creating a lean, athletic, awesome physique. I'm talking fitness magazine cover model material…NOT a huge, unnatural looking, can-barely-walk-through-the-door type of body. I'm 5ft 8ins and only weigh between 71kg-73kg, and so there are much bigger guys strolling around gyms where I live. But I'm not interested in their biceps measurements, their muscle vests, or their annoying grunting noises in the gym.

What's more important for me is that…

I'm in better shape now at 34 than I was at 20, I'm strong as hell, and I maintain lean muscle, low body fat levels and six pack abs easily. All through training for less than three hours per week.

You can achieve the same, no matter what shape you're in just now. In this book I share with you the same healthy, sustainable approach to training and diet that you can really enjoy and maintain.

Lifting heavy weights in intense training sessions, supported with proper nutrition, decent rest and stress management is the way to more muscle, less fat and the body you've probably only dreamed of.

This is the way for <u>both men and women</u>. No sexism here, women should be doing the same weightlifting exercises and going as heavy as they can too.

As for cardio – it's cancelled.

Apart from burning calories inefficiently, jogging, running, fitness classes etc have virtually no impact on muscle tone and overall body composition. I'm very much biased here but...cardio is pretty much a waste of time.

I think we all secretly know this, but persevere anyway thinking noticeable changes are just around the corner.

Let's be honest, looking in the mirror after weeks and months of trekking on the treadmill is proof that it's literally getting us nowhere. And swishing about on the elliptical machine feels like it's sucking out your soul.

Yet so many people carry with this type of mind-numbing, ineffective training – despite the lack of exercise excitement and obvious lack of results in their physique.

Strength training / weight training / barbell training...whatever you choose to call it...is a different story. It can: transform your physique in a matter of months, increase your strength, burn fat more efficiently, improve your mental health, strengthen your heart, lower your risk of disease, boost your self-esteem, prevent against injuries, improve your posture, the list goes on...

Why then do too many men and women avoid lifting weights like they should? Here's the problem:

#1 They fear they'll create a 'bulky' over-developed look.

#2 They think it involves training 5, 6 or 7 days per week.

#3 They worry it means a super strict regimented diet for the rest of their days.

#4 They're put off lifting heavy weights by the muscle vest wearing, loud grunting, selfie-taking, pill-popping, ego-maniacs they see in the gym (...and every gym in the world has their share).

Ultimately these people don't want to become a MEATHEAD.

'Meathead'? C'mon, you know what I mean. Every gym has its share of resident meatheads. Inflated bodies, inflated egos, and they reckon their training and diet way is the only way.

It's all about being better than everyone else rather *bettering themselves*.

I genuinely believe this kind of attitude and approach is what turns most people off when it comes to weight training. It's frustrating because thousands upon thousands of people across the world are missing out on the huge benefits strength training can bring.

The meathead approach to exercise and diet is fuelled by a multi-billion dollar sports supplements industry. This spews out all sorts of misinformation in fitness magazines and advertisements about what it takes to build the great body you've always wanted.

This results in another huge turn-off for people who are given the wrong impression that they must...

- Train 5,6,7 days per week.

- Guzzle whey protein shakes every day (...and feel like a bloated balloon).

- Meal prep every day (...until they become the most miserable people they know).

- Become some sort of macronutrients/macronutrients mathematician (...counting every calorie like crazy).

- Spend a fortune on supplements (...that are really a waste of money).

- Spend half the day eating small, regular meals.

This is all rubbish. You don't have to listen to all the confusing advice out there. And you don't have to worry about what any gym meathead tells you anymore because this book cuts out all the crap.

It provides you with solid strategies for building muscle, burning fat and sculpting a fantastic physique.

You'll also learn about...

- The most effective exercises for more muscle, less fat
- Proven training systems
- A framework to not only perform at the right weights level, but to also make steady progress
- A simplified formula for creating your own training programs easily
- Why lifting weights more than just 3 days per week is not only unnecessary, but can be counter-productive
- Top tactics to stay motivated and keep you on track until you get results
- Laying a solid nutritional foundation to get the most out of your efforts in the gym

I lift weights three days per week – and each session rarely exceeds one hour. Despite what you may have been told, more is definitely not better when it comes to strength training.

It's all about training smarter, not harder. This books shows you how you can gain lean muscle, incinerate fat, and realistically get in the best shape of your life....training for less than three hours per week.

I don't want that to sound like hyped-up bullsh*t...and it also doesn't mean this book is a shortcut to success. Training hard and sticking with the plan is not always easy. Nothing worth achieving truly is.

But you CAN achieve your health and fitness goals if you push yourself, stay consistent, ignore all the confusing advice out there, and stick to the sensible, healthy, do-able approach in this book.

After nearly two decades of experimentation with countless training and dietary approaches, I have a formula that works. It has been proven in my own experience and time and again with my clients.

It's all laid out in this book. It's simply up to you to implement it.

Ready to become a leaner, stronger, better version of yourself?

Let's get into this!

Chapter 1

Cutting Out the Confusion

One fitness magazine promises you "beach ready abs within three weeks"...

...while the one sitting on the shelf next to it has the "ultimate guide to bigger biceps".

Your mate in work writes down his training routine and you give that a bash. Halfway through the workout your gym's resident meathead kindly tells you it's a waste of time – and then proceeds to show you what you "really should be doing". Without you even asking.

Information overload.

When it comes to health and fitness, we're bombarded from every corner with advice on what to do. There's so much information and so many options that you probably don't know where to start.

On the other hand, you may have fallen into the trap of trying everything – and mastering nothing.

It's time to cut through the confusion and simplify weight training and diet for those looking to finally make some positive progress in changing their physique.

To do this, we'll focus on four key areas in this chapter:

- **Compound exercises**
- **Training with the right volume and intensity**
- **Proper recovery**
- **Preparation and staying motivated**

Later in the book I'll delve into these key areas even further and provide you with clear steps to take, meaning you can cut out all the confusion once and for all.

I bought the same fitness magazines you've probably picked up at some point. In fact I subscribed to two of them. In every issue there's always pages and pages filled with demonstrations of some fancy new exercises / workout routines.

Some guy in a sleeveless shirt and shiny shorts doing 23 convoluted moves on medicine balls, using ropes, or lying on the floor.

I'd try to remember all these moves (because taking the magazine into the gym with me wouldn't have been a good look). Then I'd try them out, generally feeling pretty awkward, and usually with a clumsy technique.

Most of the time I didn't really feel much benefit and, after two or three weeks, I forgot all about them. Then the next magazine came out and I was onto trying something else out.

I must've tried out over 100 different exercises I saw in these magazines and I'd say I only use just four or five of them these days. That's because most of them were a different variation on the same kind of muscle isolation exercises. Fact is: you don't really need to know 73 different ways to work your biceps.

A much better strategy is becoming great at the biggest and best exercises that have been around since the beginning. The ones that have stood the test of time. The exercises that deliver the best bang for your buck….I'm talking about **'compounds'**.

Compound Exercises

Compounds exercises are the big, bold, buster moves such as barbell squats, deadlifts and chin-ups. They are so effective for two reasons:

1. They work several muscle groups at once.
2. They stimulate an anabolic environment in the body, which equals more muscle and less fat.

Problem is – way too many gym-goers avoid doing these ultra effective weight training exercises. Why? Because they're tough.

But we've all got to start somewhere. And compounds are the way to go for anyone looking to create a lean, athletic body with great overall body composition.

<u>Therefore, the training advice in this book centres around all the key compound exercises. No matter what level you're starting at, you can become a master at these movements - and you'll make faster progress than most other gym-goers as a result.</u>

To this day, compound exercises still make up the majority of my workouts. The ratio of compound to muscle isolation exercises is roughly 75:25. While there will also be some valuable muscle isolation exercises included, we'll mainly focus on the ultra effective compound movements.

It's all about <u>efficiency</u> and <u>effectiveness</u>.

Squats, for example, target your thighs, calves, butt, abs and lower back all in one movement, while chin-ups work your biceps, forearms, shoulders, and entire upper back.

An isolation exercise, like the leg curl machine for example, works only the quadriceps.

What would you rather do? Spend two hours in the gym, jumping from machine to machine, and doing around 20 different muscle isolation exercises in the hope you've worked your entire body?

Or – spend 45-60 minutes focusing intently on 6-7 big compound movements that force several muscle groups to work together...in a manner that leaves you in no doubt you've smashed your training session?

And no, it ain't just powerlifters or bodybuilders who do the likes of squats, deadlifts and bench pressing.

It's the clued-up men and women who realise that compounds can:

- Stimulate muscle growth AND fat loss more effectively than other exercises.
- Help them sculpt an athletic, well defined physique instead of a 'bulky' look.
- See their strength gains go through the roof.
- Make their training much more exciting than ever before.

From what I've seen in gyms over the years, a high percentage of people always miss out the squats, deadlifts etc. To me this is crazy.

This is where following the advice in this book you'll be ahead of the game.

In chapter three, we'll go into much more detail about compounds - and using them properly to your full advantage.

Training Volume and Intensity

You know that phrase, 'go hard or go home'? It sounds a bit cringey, but unless you're actually lifting heavy and hitting it hard in the gym you might aswell be at home. It's time to turn the volume up when it comes to your training.

Lifting heavier weights with fewer reps targets the 'fast twitch' muscle fibres. These are required for power and strength. Progressively overloading the muscles with more weight also triggers myofibrillar hypertrophy – which is essentially your muscles developing in strength and size in response to this form of heavy training.

"But how heavy is heavy...?"

"How many reps are enough to kickstart muscle building...?"

"Am I doing enough sets of the exercises to actually get results...?"

Just some of the questions I hear from my online personal training clients. (I choose to do web-based personal training as it means I can work with people from all over the world – and it empowers them to get results without me holding their hand in the gym).

Working Out Using The 3, 6, 9 Principle

Introducing my 3, 6, 9 Principle which ensure you're training with the right volume and intensity.

Number of sets....3 is sufficient.

How heavy....6 is the minimum number of reps you must be able to complete with a particular weight.

Muscle building....9 is the maximum number of reps you want to reach before taking training to the next level through progressive overload.

Varying your training routine is extremely important and this will also achieved in terms of mixing up different exercises, the order you complete them, rest periods between sets etc.

However, applying The 3,6,9 Principle gives you solid markers for sets, minimum amount of reps, and a clear indication of when you're ready to move on to the next level. This will ensure you make the best progress in the gym.

Proper Recovery – Real Results Come Outside Of The Gym

The idea of lifting weights 5, 6, 7 days per week in order to get in great shape like any good Meathead would do probably ain't that appealing to you.

That's fine – because you don't have to.

What if I told you that just three heavy weights sessions per week was enough training to build muscle and burn fat effectively?

Training nearly every day of the week is not necessary. In some cases it can actually be counter-productive and lead to injury.

The body requires sufficient rest to repair the damage done to muscle tissue during intense weight training. Many weightlifters get round this by working specific muscle groups on certain days.

But this is not necessary either. By working various muscle groups at once using compound exercises you ensure a total body workout. And if you're training properly at a high level of intensity, as described in this book, then you'll need a day's rest in between workouts.

When it comes to your training week, more is not always better. We're going for quality over quantity. That means:

* Focusing on the biggest and best exercises (aka compounds)

* Lifting heavy and progressively overloading the weight

* Making every single rep count

* Working so intensely that you need one day on, one day off, to properly recover

The inevitable and unavoidable DOMS (delayed onset muscle soreness) from training this way should be enough to convince you that it makes complete sense to lift weights just 3 or 4 days per week.

Proper rest and recovery is too often overlooked in the health and fitness industry. People are so desperate to see results tomorrow that they continue to hit the weights hard even when their body is still patching up the damage from the previous session.

This puts the brakes on progress. To realise this, you must understand the basic science of lifting weights, coupled with healthy nutrition, in order to build muscle and burn fat.

The type of training we'll be doing - lifting heavy weights with lower reps - causes tiny tears on the muscle fibres. This shocks the muscles into *myofibrillar hypertrophy* – which essentially leads to your muscle fibres growing bigger and stronger to try and adapt to the weightlifting strain.

This growth process really kicks in after you've finished your last rep in the gym. In order to maximise the gains from our workouts we must give the body the tools it needs to repair those muscle fibre tears (i.e. healthy, nutritious food) – and get enough rest for the job to be done properly without more strain on the muscles.

That's why, following the training advice in this book, 3-4 days of strength training is sufficient for building muscle and burning fat effectively. And efficiently.

Preparation And Staying Motivated

Preparing properly and staying motivated go hand in hand. Problem is, most of us miss out the preparation part.

Can you remember the last time you tried to gain muscle, develop six-pack abs, or lose the layer of flab that just wouldn't shift?

It's usually in January with a New Year's resolution...or about six weeks before we go on holiday! We get all fired up about making it happen 'this time'. Buy new gym shoes, stock on up healthy food, think positive thoughts about the lean, muscular version of you.

You convince a friend to start hitting the gym with you, and you set about training with a full tank of will-power. The first session was tough but you're determined this time.

Fast forward 3-4 weeks...

You've got so much going on at work right now. By the time you get to the gym after work it'll be so late you'll probably only have about 30 minutes max to train. Plus, your friend skipped the last two sessions and probably won't make it today either. Have you even got any healthy food in the fridge to cook a decent post-workout meal? *"I'll just train tomorrow..."* you tell yourself as that tank of will-power gets down to its last drop.

Let's be honest, we've all experienced this kind of scenario, or at least come up with some of these excuses. No matter how motivated you are at the beginning, it can be a real struggle for all of us to stick to our training goals. Sh*t happens.

But through proper preparation we can avoid giving into excuses and going completely off track. There are tricks and tools we can use to supercharge our motivation, prevent our willpower from wilting, and stick with the plan until we start seeing results.

That's what the next chapter is all about.

CHECKLIST

* Step back from 'information overload' – and focus solely on the 'non-meathead' approach to building muscle and burning fat.

* You don't have to know how to perform countless exercises, or the latest fitness fad routine.

* Compound weight training exercises are the most effective and efficient ways of building muscle and burning fat.

* Compound exercises work various muscle groups at once – and create an anabolic environment in the body. This means more muscle and less fat.

* It's time to turn up the volume in your training: lifting heavy with fewer reps.

* Use The 3,6,9 Principle to make solid progress in your training: 3 sets, no fewer than 6 reps, and add more weight as soon as you can hit 9 reps.

* You DON'T have to train 5,6,7 days per week.

* Lifting weights 3-4 days per week can deliver outstanding results when it comes to building muscle and burning fat.

* One day on, one day off lifting weights is ideal because our body requires proper rest to repair damage to muscle fibres. This recovery period assists in muscle growth following intense training sessions.

* Proper preparation is crucial to staying motivated and to avoid going off track.

Chapter 2

Preparation and Goal Setting For Maximum Results

Picture this...

You hit the gym with real confidence because you have a masterplan. Clear, defined goals for once. And you're finally focusing on the right exercises.

So no more worrying if you're doing enough in your workouts to build muscle.

No more wandering about the gym and simply jumping on whatever machine is free.

You have focus – and <u>that focus alone sparks real motivation</u>.

The post-workout soreness and <u>surprising gains in strength</u> after just a handful of workouts has another positive knock-on effect...

You don't need as much willpower to stick to a healthy diet. Junk food just ain't as appealing when you're clearly making steady progress, even at this early stage.

Buzzing for every upcoming weights session, you start hitting personal bests you thought you never had in you.

"You Start Seeing Some Proper Muscle Definition..."

Remember when the gym used to be boring? Remember when you were always fighting the excuses to miss a session? Not now.

For the first time you start seeing some proper muscle definition and your posture naturally changes. You hold yourself upwards more confidently.

This confidence you've quietly nurtured through a commitment to becoming a stronger, healthier you then gradually filters into your relationships with other people, your career, other sports etc.

Why? **You may only be lifting heavy weights, but ultimately you're bettering yourself.** This is then surprisingly reflected in other places outside of the gym.

It feels amazing when people start commenting on the difference in your physique.

That spurs you on even further, but at this stage who needs motivation now anyway?

What feels even better is the rush of endorphins bursting out of your head after every workout.

<u>You're a stronger, fitter, healthier, leaner, better version of you</u>.

If you're just starting out, or if you've been training for years but got nowhere, then you won't be familiar with the above scenario.

But this IS how your body and health transformation can unfold for you. I've experienced it myself and witnessed it with clients.

All you have to do is follow the advice in this book – and apply it.

Two Things That Are the Difference Between Failure and Success

The first crucial step in this chain of events leading to a stronger, healthier, better you is proper preparation and goal setting.

These build solid foundations for success – and are the difference between quitting and actually getting somewhere.

This is essential. Failing to prepare is preparing to fail. (I've clearly ripped off someone's cliché here, but it's true).

Getting this right at the beginning means you'll be fully focused and prepared so that you stick with the programme long enough to begin to see results.

Once those results come you're given even more juice to keep going to start making more progress. Others start noticing the difference and then you're HOOKED. You won't have to read this chapter again, the need for willpower will dwindle – and your motivation levels will naturally be elevated.

Preparing For Success

Everyone who takes up strength training, or any other form of exercise, to get in great shape all have one thing in common: we do it as a reaction to something.

For me, it was simply a cheeky comment about my "skinny arms" in front a big group of people. Aged 16 and very self-conscious about my weak, thin body, I felt humiliated and this anger was enough to kickstart my hobby/healthy obsession with weight training.

Someone may have made a thoughtless throw-away comment about your weight and it hit you hard.

Maybe you're getting married in six months and are worried about not looking your best in your wedding photos.

Whatever you're reacting to sparks enough motivation to get started - in that moment.

Problem is, that fuel runs out fairly soon <u>if you haven't prepared properly</u>. You see it in every gym across the world every year.

Gym memberships skyrocket in January due to New Year resolutions and plenty of good intentions...

People don't prepare properly or stick to a plan....

They get bored because they don't see immediate results...

Gym population returns to normal by mid-February, most of the new faces have disappeared.

You wouldn't run a marathon without properly preparing first, would you? Same goes for lifting weights and transforming your body.

You're not going to be able to achieve a chiselled physique overnight, but you can definitely achieve it – and preparing properly will give you a firm foundation to build upon.

Five Principle Pieces of Preparation

#1 Gym membership

I might be stating the obvious here but this point is for the benefit of anyone considering buying a dumbbell set and lifting at home, or working out in your garage. Don't waste your time or money because you simply won't make enough progress.

It's absolutely essential that you join a local gym that has all the correct equipment to support the type of exercises and workout programs I discuss later in chapter 4.

Also, you'll experience a rapid gain in strength by following the advice laid out in this book. You would outgrow your home weights in no time and, if you don't move on to the next level, then neither will your results.

#2 Setting goals

This is the part that most people miss out – and is one of the main reasons we see all those new faces at the gym in January and never see them again after February.

With clear, defined goals you'll:

- Have a target to aim for
- Be inspired to get going
- Put some real meaning behind your workouts
- Be MUCH less likely to quit

Without clear, defined goals you'll:

- Get bored easily and look for excuses
- Have no real perception of progress

- End up majorly frustrated
- Run out of motivation quickly
- Undoubtedly quit and end up back at square one

We'll discuss goals further and how to set them properly soon.

#3 Gym training diary

Using a gym training diary is one of the simplest, yet most powerful pieces of advice I could give you. A cheap, small pocket sized diary transformed my workouts in various ways – and this can have a huge impact on your progress too.

Do you get bored easily or struggle to keep pushing forward when training on your own? Or do you sometimes forget what you lifted last time round and therefore don't have a clue if you're making progress?

Well, a training journal solves these problems and should be your body's Bible for the following reasons:

- Laser sharp focus.

To help you stay focused it's extremely important you map out the workout ahead and set goals. Don't worry about what anyone else is lifting, we're not interested in them.

By writing down exactly what you plan to achieve in the gym in advance you're much less likely to be distracted by anything else. It also gives you a definitive plan and targets to aim for, giving your workouts even more purpose.

- Accountability.

When you step into the gym your training session should be all about continuous personal improvement – and setting new personal bests. It doesn't matter if you don't have a training partner. You have the training journal to answer to!

It's there to record your score for every exercise – and for some reason that small pile of paper holds you to account. It's your training partner that can't talk. It can tell you how far you have progressed. It reminds you of exactly how you performed last time around. And it can guilt trip you into doing even better this time.

- Better performance.

A training journal means your workout plan is there in front of you in black and white. So, there's no skipping the last couple of exercises because then you'll have to leave that part blank - or score the exercises out completely - when filling in your training journal.

Then the next time you're training you'll be reminded of how you cheated yourself last time around. See what I mean about the guilt trips?

This naturally makes you want to complete ALL the exercises listed in your journal – and squeeze out a rep or two more than you thought you could.

- Staying on Track

As you become stronger and continually take your training to the next level, you'll be surprised how hard it is trying to remember the level of weights you reached or number of reps you completed for all the various exercises you're doing every week.

Our usual response to this: default to the lighter weight. This means you're not pushing yourself hard enough and are missing out on gains.

- Motivation

As that journal starts filling up with performances you didn't think you had in you, it will fire you up big time. Seeing those weightlifting numbers climb as the weeks go past gives you an extra injection of motivation.

You'll know for certain you're making progress because it's there in black and white. That gives you more confidence, gets you buzzing for your next workout, and automatically provides the motivation you previously struggled to find.

- Sense of Achievement

And finally…the rush of endorphins usually makes us feel great after a tough workout, but this is enhanced when you see on paper everything you have just put your body through.

And flicking through your notes, seeing where you have started and how far you have come, is amazingly satisfying.

#4 Scheduling your training a week in advance

Another problem that sinks good intentions and derails many health and fitness programs is being vague.

We've all told ourselves at some point, *"I'm going to make the gym three or four times per week"*. Let's be honest, it usually doesn't take very long before life takes over and we're only managing to train a couple of days per week.

Then we beat ourselves up, lose motivation and quit.

The perfect solution to this is to schedule your workouts a week in advance in your new training diary.

It need only take 20 minutes on a Sunday. First, analyse your working week and identify the days and <u>exact times</u> you can work out.

Pinpoint four training slots – and make them non-negotiable. Fit your day around them, instead of the other way round.

#5 Stock up on the right foods

We're in the game of sculpting a brand new lean, athletic, ripped physique. Weight training is the sculptor – and the right foods are his tools.

There are three main reasons why we must clear the junk out of our cupboards and fill up on unprocessed, whole foods.

1. Proper nutrition before training will help fuel your workouts.

2. The nutrients they provide give your body what it needs after lifting heavy weights to repair tissue damage and build muscle.

3. It will boost your immune system and improve your overall health.

We've got pretty tough workouts coming up and a quarter pounder meal ain't gonna help us get through it.

And just because KFC sells chicken doesn't mean we should make a detour there on the way home from the gym either.

Seriously, we want to make the most of our gym efforts. We can do that by supporting our body's transformation with proper nutrition.

Fortunately, that doesn't mean being on some sort of crazy diet that makes you miserable...and you eventually end up quitting anyway. No, the dietary advice in this book is do-able, sensible and definitely achievable.

We'll serve up plenty on diet in chapter 8, but for now bear in mind that clearing out most of the junk and stocking up on healthy foods is another essential piece of preparation.

The Power Of Goal Setting

"Set a goal to achieve something that is so big, so exciting that is excites you and scares you at the same time." – Bob Proctor.

All the hugely successful people in this world usually have two things in common:

1. 1 – They are physically fit because they know that looking after their bodies will also sharpen their minds.

2. 2 – They set goals and go about achieving them with a laser like focus.

Goal setting is very important before you lift a single dumbbell because it clears the path leading to where you want to be and gives you targets to zero in on.

By writing down your body transformation goals down and keeping them in mind, it prevents you from training aimlessly, spurs you on - and plays a big role in keeping you on track.

There are three key elements to setting powerful goals.

#1 Be specific about what you want – and aim high

We don't do vague goals like, 'I want more muscle', or 'I want to lose my belly fat'. That's hardly inspiring, is it?

Specific details about your perfect body is more like it. No point in setting the bar low, let's raise it right up and get fired up about the possibility of completely transforming your physique.

Think about how achieving this will make you *feel*.

#2 Set your starting point

To get where we're going we need to know where we are. Take measurements, date, weight, size of waist, arms etc.

Also, take a 'before' picture. Nobody really likes doing this as it feels awkward, but it will feel much better looking at it when you have the 'after' photo to compare it to.

#3 Set a deadline

Choose a date – between 12 and 16 weeks from now – and make that your deadline for hitting your goals.

This is the ideal period because if the deadline is too far in the distance you'll slack off. We want a sense of urgency as we chase these goals.

CHECKLIST

* Proper preparation and goal setting are the difference between quitting too soon and getting results.

* Don't lift weights at home or in your garage because your progress will be limited. Join your local gym instead.

* Use a gym training diary to properly keep track of your progress, boost motivation and help you stay on track.

* Plan your three gym workouts a week in advance - and keep those important appointments with yourself.

* Clear the junk foods out of your cupboards, so there's less room for temptation.

* Write down your weight training goals – and make them specific and detailed.

* Take all the relevant weight/body measurements, and a 'before' picture, to ensure you have a clear starting point.

* Set a deadline – 12-16 weeks is an ideal time frame – for hitting your goals.

Chapter 3

The Secret To Staying On Track

Do you get bored at the gym sometimes? A struggle to drag yourself in there after a long day at work? Then you leave knowing your session was only a half-hearted effort...

We've all been there. Training without a partner was another problem for me in the past, I just never got as much out of working out on my own.

These are all just tiny barriers on the road to success and can easily be overcome.

The secret to staying on track is by...

#1 Not changing everything at once

Right now we're planning, preparing and getting in the right mindset for building a new body. Later there will be clear instructions on training and advice on diet, nutrition and rest.

Taking all of this on board, particularly when it comes to diet and rest, might mean a complete lifestyle change for you. Trying to implement everything at once to achieve your goals will lead to overwhelm and frustration.

The answer - don't change everything at once. In my 12 week programme with personal training clients, we introduce one positive habit per week primarily with nutrition, i.e. cut your sugar intake by half, or have a takeaway meal just at the weekend, rather than 2 or 3 days per week.

We build upon each weekly habit and it all adds up to major shifts and great results.

It's much easier to stick with gradual changes rather than turning your entire life upside down. Sticking to the same healthy task each day for the whole week helps to naturally form positive habits. Soon it isn't so difficult to stick to them.

#2 Treat your training diary as your body's Bible – and fill it in religiously

Writing in this little book might seem trivial, maybe even pointless to some people, but planning your workouts and keeping record of your performance will supercharge your progress. Trust me.

A training diary gives you focus, accountability, improves your performance, keeps you on track, motivated and heightens your sense of achievement.

The coaches at Crossfit Los Angeles have made it a requirement that every one of their clients keeps a training journal. It's because they know how powerful it is in bringing the best out of people and achieving amazing results.

I know from experience that if I've not planned out my workouts in advance, or if I've left my training journal at home, then I always have a mediocre workout. And mediocre training equals mediocre results.

#3 Review your goals daily

Write down your clear, defined goals and make it a habit to spend just 30 seconds reading them every morning.

Keep reminding yourself of what you intend to achieve and how you're going to feel once you do it.

It's a simple habit but one that keeps you focused on your targets and bats any excuses right out of the park.

If They Can Do It So Can You…

Too often we limit ourselves mentally when it comes to what we want to achieve. That's why I emphasised that when you set your goals make sure you aim high.

It doesn't matter where you are just now. Whether you think you're too skinny and weak, too fat, unhealthy, not athletic enough, don't have the right genes, or whatever other crazy thought process enters your head.

These are all just limiting beliefs. They may have held you back until now, but they hold no real weight.

There are some amazing people out there who prove that once you set a firm intention with the mind, the body will follow suit. At the time of writing, check out what these superhero pensioners were achieving…

Danish weightlifter Svend Stensgaard deadlifts 290lbs and says the rush of endorphins he gets from lifting weights is like a "dosage of morphine".

<u>Svend is 97 years old</u> at the time of writing this and is the world's oldest powerlifter.

New York supergran Willie Murphy weighs just 105lbs but she trains like a boss in the gym – and has got the biceps to prove it.

Aged 78, Willie can do one-handed push-ups and pull-ups – and deadlifts double her own bodyweight.

Pat Reeves has beaten cancer twice – through a raw foods diet only and lifting weights to strengthen her body.

Aged 71, she's the UK's oldest competing female powerlifter, and has some words of wisdom for us: "Be pro-active, find a goal/dream and every day do something that progresses you towards that.

"Be clear about what you want, not just aiming to 'improve' but being exactly specific as to projected achievement."

These people are the inspiration that you CAN significantly improve the condition of your body and your overall health – no matter your level of fitness right now.

Time to get started.

CHECKLIST

- If you don't already have a gym membership, sign up for an induction at your local gym.

- Buy yourself a gym training diary for scheduling your workouts and designing your training programme using the exercises and systems described later in chapter 4.

- Write down your clear, detailed goals.

Chapter 4

Building Muscle and Burning Fat Through Compound Exercises

A few years ago I used to see the same guy in the gym virtually every time I went, whether I arrived at 4.30pm, 5pm, 6.08pm. I'm still wondering if he was paying rent!

He lifted weights but would jump from machine to machine, sometimes going back to the same one 20 minutes later.

But not once did I see him squat. Never did I see him do deadlifts, or clean and press.

After one gym workout I overheard him talking to another guy in the locker room and he said: "Glad that's over. That was two and a half hours today."

The other guy replied: "That's a serious gym session!"

He said: "I was in for three hours on Sunday."

Fair play to the guy for showing up and putting in the work – but it was getting him nowhere. I saw him in the gym constantly for a solid six months and never noticed any change in his physique.

This was because he was making several mistakes. Firstly – he was judging his workouts based on the amount of time he spent in the gym. Focusing on the correct exercises and training at the right intensity is far more important than how many minutes you've been sweating.

Secondly – he was training inefficiently doing countless muscle isolation exercises, with no real structure to his workouts or system in place for progressing to the next level.

Pretty sure I saw him make a pit-stop at Burger King on the way home too....

Seriously, we can completely wipe out these same mistakes and guarantee muscle gains by placing a huge emphasis on compound exercises, training at the right intensity and optimising our diet.

Compound exercises are the most <u>effective</u> and <u>efficient</u> way of training.

I'm crazy about compounds. Within a few weeks of hitting them hard you will be too. Why?

Because you'll finally know what it's like to work your body properly and feel every muscle ache afterwards.

You'll witness your strength go through the roof.

And you'll see clear results in your physique as gradually gain muscle and strip away fat (...provided you don't make a detour to Burger King too after your workouts).

Now we're ready to really get down to business.

Time to introduce the top 10 compound movements our training will centre around, along with a selection of effective muscle isolation exercises that will be weaved into our workouts too.

Proper technique is crucial so there are clear written instructions on how to perform each move correctly, along with tips on common mistakes to avoid.

Also listed are the muscles worked in each exercise – which will underline exactly how effective compound exercises are for achieving a total body workout and creating optimal body composition.

Why Compound Exercises Build Muscle AND Burn Fat

Heavy weight training using compound exercises – particularly squats and deadlifts – has been scientifically proven to boost production of anabolic hormones, growth hormone and testosterone. (Don't worry ladies, this isn't a problem for you as your testosterone levels are naturally 15-20 times lower than men).

- Testosterone is the primary hormone that interacts with muscle tissue, repairing the tiny tears caused during heavy lifting and stimulating development.

- Growth hormone is also a main player in muscle growth because it enhances uptake of amino acids (the building blocks of protein) and protein synthesis in muscle. At the same time, it also increases lipolysis (fat breakdown) and the use of fatty acids by the body. So, it's a two for one with GH – more muscle and less fat.

Creating this anabolic environment in the body leads to hypertrophy – growth in the size of muscle cells.

It's the combination of heavy lifting and large groups of muscle involved that sparks this process. Other forms of exercise simply don't have the same muscle building effect.

Gaining Muscle Is Like Adding More Coal To A Fat Burning Fire

To maintain muscle your body burns more calories than it does holding on to fat.

Some experts estimate that each extra pound of muscle burns an additional 30-50 calories per day.

Ultimately, it's beneficial for your metabolism to gain muscle mass. Just by developing muscle, your body naturally becomes more efficient at burning fat.

Muscle gain and fat loss go hand in hand.

Other Benefits Of Compound Exercises

#1 Several muscle groups are worked at once

Why do three or four leg machine exercises when you can get the same benefits, and more, from barbell squats? The nature of compounds is that they engage several muscle groups in one complete movement. This is what makes them so efficient.

#2 Better body composition

We've all seen the Johnny Bravo type physiques. Gym goers with a puffed-out chest, broad shoulders – and legs like twigs. Too much muscle isolation work can result in specific body parts being over-developed, although this isn't too common. By working various muscle groups in a synergistic way, compound exercises avoid this and sculpt a natural athletic physique.

#3 Improves heart health

The short intense nature of compound exercises also work the cardiovascular system effectively. It's not all about building muscle and burning fat, compounds are good for your ticker too.

#4 You can complete your workouts quicker

To achieve a total body workout and fatigue your muscles enough to spark muscle growth, you could do upwards of a dozen different muscle isolation exercises. With compounds hitting various muscle groups at once, you could achieve the same end goal using just half the amount of exercises. That means less time spent in the gym unnecessarily.

#5 Rapid gains in strength

By forcing different muscle groups to 'pull together' to deal with the strain of whatever compound exercise you're engaging in you'll surprisingly gain strength rapidly. By working out applying The 3,6,9 Principle you'll likely make huge strength strides in a matter of weeks, which will of course lead to muscle gain.

#6 Every squat adds a day to your life!

Still can't find the scientific study proving this one - you're just gonna have to trust me on it!

Gaining Muscle And Burning Fat – But At The Same Time?

Most fitness professionals will tell you that you can't build muscle and burn fat effectively at the same time. That you either have to shed the pounds and then work on gaining muscle afterwards, or that you need to 'bulk' then 'cut'.

I disagree. I've seen people achieve it, and there are experts out there who have helped folk achieve both goals at once.

In a recent interview with Bodybuilding.com, Stephen Adele, fitness coach, best-selling author and owner of nutritional firm iSatori, argued that it's inaccurate to say it's impossible to build muscle and lose bodyfat at the same time. The fitness firm boss says it's all down to your approach and described such a double success as a "true transformation".

The approach to training within the next few chapters are exactly what you need to help you achieve both muscle gain and fat loss.

"But what if I've tried compound exercises before and I got nowhere?", some readers might ask.

There are two more important elements to achieving this muscle gain/fat loss body transformation. Miss any of them out and you won't get the results you want. They are:

1. Not coupling your training with a <u>healthy, whole foods diet</u>, and breaking some of the foundational nutrition rules.

2. Not being <u>consistent</u> with either training or diet.

You CAN Achieve Amazing Results...But Nothing Worth Having Comes Easy

Another question you might ask is, "How long is this all going to take?"

I wrote an article a few months ago for The Good Men Project website titled, '11 Mistakes Every Gym Rookie Makes'. Number 11 on that list was 'not being consistent' because the problem with most people is that they don't stick with the programme long enough to see any results.

We now live in the 21st century where it's all about instant gratification. We text somebody - and we're annoyed if we don't get a reply within 10 minutes!

Don't be a gym rookie.

I know you're taking your plan to build muscle and burn fat much more seriously than that anyway...simply by the fact that you've bought this book.

Nothing really worth having comes easy. Same goes for that awesome physique you've been chasing. It won't come overnight, or over a fortnight, but you CAN achieve amazing results if you're consistent with your training and following a healthy diet.

You can't put a number on something like this because our bodies are all different, with various compositions, fat levels, bone density, rates of metabolism etc, so your body transformation is not something you can accurately schedule.

Having said that, I'd still expect most people to start seeing a positive difference in their body shape – and overall health and wellbeing – within 4-6 weeks, provided they stick with the advice on training and diet.

One of my recent online personal training clients, Chris Hannan, lost 10lbs in just 10 days. The 33-year-old father-of-one is now taking his body transformation to the next level and so can you.

CHECKLIST

* Compound exercises are the most effective and efficient way of training.

* Heavy weight training using compound exercises, particularly squats and deadlifts, have been proven to boost the production of muscle building anabolic hormones.

* Other forms of training, like standard cardio and endurance training, simply does not have the same effect in developing a great body.

* More muscle = more calories burned naturally.

* It's estimated that your body uses an extra 30-50 calories to maintain each additional pound of muscle you gain.

* Other benefits of compounds include: several muscle groups worked at once, better body composition, improved heart health, a total body workout, and rapid gains in strength.

* Don't listen to the naysayers – you CAN build muscle and burn fat at the same time.

* Results won't come overnight, but they will come – if you stay consistent with your training and diet.

Chapter 5

Compound Exercises: Bigger Movements, Better Results

I'm always banging on about compound exercises and these are the top moves I believe everyone should be doing whether you're a man, woman...or reptile.

Looking to build lean muscle? Develop definition? Strip fat?

These 10 exercises will form the core of your training, along with some muscle isolation moves I'll introduce in the next chapter.

I give descriptions of each exercise but it's too tricky to include high quality photos in this book, particularly the Kindle version. But I want to make sure you get the most from this book and I realise some readers might not be familiar with some of the exercises at all, so I've created an exercise demo guide that you can download for free on my website.

It includes high quality pictures of me performing all 25 exercises...(and pulling some weird looking faces during them). You can download it for free on my website via the web address below (I've included the link at the end of this book too).

www.weighttrainingistheway.com/exercise-demos

#1 Barbell Squats

The King of exercises – and one to master if you're serious about building muscle, losing fat, and changing the way you look and feel.

Technique

>> Warm up for a couple of minutes doing a light jog on a treadmill and then a series of leg stretches.

>> Place the barbell on the squat rack at shoulder height and add the weight plates to each side. Ensure they are locked on using a collar or clamp. Also put safety bars in place just below waist height (as seen in the picture).

>> Position yourself under the centre of the bar so that it sits on your trapezius. Stretch your hands out and grip the bar at either side at a length that feels comfortable.

>> Lift the bar upwards off the hooks and step back with both feet.

>> Position your feet in a natural standing position, toes pointing forward and slightly outwards.

>> Keep your back rigid, holding the barbell on your trapezius with good posture.

>> Staring straight ahead, squat down in a controlled manner until your thighs are parallel with the floor or just slightly lower.

>> Keeping your eyesight focused ahead, push back up forcefully through your hips and straighten your legs back into the starting position.

Common mistakes – and how to avoid them

Arching your back during the movement. Concentrate on keeping your back rigid throughout and also keep your gaze focused on an object directly ahead as you lower yourself and until you return to the top again. This is good for balance and staying focused.

Moving your feet. Once you step back from the rack and you're in a comfortable starting position your feet should not move from that spot. Your heels may occasionally lift off the ground as you push upwards with the weight. Do not let this become a habit because it can make you unsteady. Your feet should be planted in the same position until the final rep is done.

Forgetting to lock the weights on to the bar. I've done this a few times and seen weights slide right off the bar. Always think safety first and by put a collar/clamp on the bar to make sure weights stay safely in place.

Muscles worked: The *entire lower body, particularly the quadriceps, hamstrings, glutes and calves, abs, erector spinae (group of back) muscles.*

#2 Deadlifts

Another monster move that involves multiple muscles in the upper and lower body.

The deadlift basically involves lifting a heavy weight off the floor and then standing with your legs straight and shoulders back. This one can be tricky though so make sure you start off with a light weight and pay close attention to the information below.

Technique

>> Stand at a loaded barbell with your feet slightly wider than shoulder width. Bend down and grab the bar with one hand over the top and the other underneath.

>> The grip should be just at the outside of your feet and your palms must be facing in different directions.

>> With your feet firmly on the floor and the bar close to your shins, pull the bar upwards over your knees. As you rise, push your hips forward and straighten your back.

>> The bar should be resting against your thighs as you stand straight with your shoulder pressed back. (It should always be kept close to your body throughout the exercise).

>> Bend your knees as you carefully lower the weight back down over your legs to the floor.

<u>Common mistakes to avoid</u>

Don't round your back. Keep it rigid and by looking straight ahead, rather than on the floor, helps achieve this.

Don't hitch or jerk the bar upwards. It should be lifted in one flowing, continuous movement.

Don't tip your feet forward – or move them at all – during the movement. There's a fair chance you'll end up faceplanting.

Muscles worked: Glutes, quads, hamstrings, calves, traps, (lower back), (forearms), shoulders, abs, (obliques)

#3 Bench press

The number one exercise for developing your chest muscles, especially when it comes to adding mass. The bench can be set at an incline level to focus more on the upper section of your chest, or decline to hit the lower part.

<u>Technique</u>

>> Lie on a bench under a weights rack with your feet flat on the floor. The barbell should be roughly level with your nose. Your hands should grip the bar slightly beyond shoulder width.

>> Lift off the rack and lower to the mid-section of your chest in a controlled manner.

>> Push back up forcefully and lock out your arms.

>> The first lowering part will take roughly a couple of seconds, but pushing to the top should take only half the time.

Common mistakes to avoid

Too narrow grip. This works the triceps and puts less strain on the chest. It'll also make the bar more difficult to balance, meaning you will struggle to cope with the same level of weight.

Too wide grip. This works a smaller portion of your chest and brings the shoulders more into play. A wider grip also makes the bar more unsteady and harder to balance.

Raising your lower back off the bench. There may be a very slight raise when you first lift the bar off the rack at the start of your set, but don't arch your back throughout as this will inevitably lead to injury.

Muscles worked: Pecs, anterior deltoids (front of shoulders), triceps.

#4 Clean and press

I nicknamed this one 'busters' a long time ago – because you feel absolutely busted after them! Works both the upper and lower body, which is obviously great for overall composition, but it also works the cardiovascular system hard. After one punishing set of these you'll feel like you've been running for an hour.

The clean and press basically involves lifting a barbell off the floor, hiking the weight up and pressing directly above your head.

Technique:

>> Same starting positioning for a bent over row. Stand over the bar with your back straight at a 45 degree angle.

>> Overhand grip for both hands, slightly beyond shoulder width, and with your knees tucked in between your arms.

>> Sweep the bar upwards, pushing forcefully through your hips almost in a jumping motion...but keep your feet on the floor.

>> As the barbell reaches your chest, flick your wrists so that your palms are now under the bar.

>> Then, without pausing, press the bar straight up until your arms lock out at the elbows.

>> Bring the weight down to chest again, and then bend the knees as you lower it to the floor in a controlled fashion.

Common mistakes

Arching your back at the beginning of the exercise. Your back should be at a straight 45 degree angle as you lean over to pick up the bar. Otherwise you're in danger of hurting your lower back.

Stumbling forwards or backwards during the exercise. You should be steady and the weight should be under control in one flowing movement.

Dropping the weight on to the floor. It's unsafe to just drop or throw the barbell down once you have raised it above your head. You should control the weight as you lower it to the floor and your muscles will still be working as you do so.

Muscles worked: Glutes, quads, hamstrings, traps, front shoulders, triceps, forearms.

#5 Bent over row

Want a V-shaped torso? Then do not miss this exercise out. Bent over rows work the entire upper back – and your biceps.

It's also definitely the number one exercise for developing the lats to taper the back and give it a natural, athletic look.

Technique

>> With a loaded barbell on the floor, stand with your feet just beyond shoulder width.

>> Bend the knees and grab the bar. Keep your lower back arched, chest puffed out and look straight ahead.

>> Lift the bar to your lower chest, making sure you keep the static position and don't swing up and down.

>> The bar should be brought up hard and fast, but should it should take twice the time to lower the bar under control.

Common mistakes

Straight legs during the lift. This makes the move awkward and increases your chances of injury so keep your knees bent slightly throughout.

Moving upwards during the lift. After initially lifting the bar from the floor, keep your hips in place and your upper body static. This works your upper back harder, and means you are not compensating by using your hips or lower back to help lift the weight.

Muscles worked: Lats, traps, biceps, front and rear shoulders.

#6 Upright row

The upright row of course works several muscles like the other compounds, but it primarily hits the upper trapezius. This creates the nice sloping look from your upper neck down to your shoulders. I personally saw a noticeable difference in development within a fortnight of first using this exercise.

Technique:

Note: an Ez-bar (pictured) is preferable to a straight barbell for this exercise because it allows for a full range of movement and causes less strain on your wrists.

>> Grab the loaded barbell at the two dipped points and have it resting at your knees.

>> Keeping your back straight, pull firmly upwards to just under your chin, with your elbows extending outwards.

>> Lower the bar in a controlled, slow fashion.

Common mistakes

Lifting the bar only to your chest. This is only half a rep, you must lift higher right up to your chin...without smacking yourself in the face.

Swinging your body to lift the weight. Your legs and back must be kept straight throughout to target the right muscles and stay injury free.

Muscles worked: Traps, middle of shoulders, biceps.

#7 Chin-ups

Chin-ups blast your biceps, lats, lower traps, forearms...and abs aswell while we're at it. The chin-up is a variation of the pull-up. In fact, some people switch the names about because they are so similar.

The difference between the chin-up is that your palms face inward and you have a narrower grip on the bar. This brings the biceps more into play.

Both exercises are outstanding for developing upper body strength – but most people struggle to perform even one full rep. (Don't worry, there's a clever tactic you can use to gradually build your strength on these that will eventually get you to the point where you can rattle them out easily).

Technique

>> Reach up and grab the bar above with your palms facing inwards. Your hands should be exactly shoulder width apart.

>> Pull yourself upwards and, just like pull-ups, cross your legs as they come off the floor.

>> Squeeze your biceps to pull your chin over the top of the bar.

>> Lower your body to the starting position in a controlled manner.

Common mistakes

Not lowering your body far enough. We're not interested in half reps. Lower your body right down, lock your arms out at the elbow and drag yourself back to the top.

Spreading your hands too far across the bar. This makes the move awkward, putting strain on your shoulders and chest which could result in injury – or falling.

Not climbing high enough. For a full rep your chin must at least touch the bar, if not go slightly over it.

Muscles worked: Lats, biceps, lower traps, forearms, abs.

- Chin-ups and the next exercise pull-ups are so good for developing your upper body, but they're very difficult at first and most people struggle to do even one rep.

- But don't just give up on these amazing exercises – you can do assisted reps until you develop enough upper body strength and/or lose bodyfat if you need to.

Some gyms have a machine you can rest your knees on which is ideal for assisting people in doing chin-ups, pull-ups and dips. If your gym doesn't have one of these then I'd highly recommend investing in a resistance band. These serve the same purpose, taking some of the load of your bodyweight while you do the exercise.

Once you can comfortably do 10 chin-ups, pull-ups or dips using the band then you'll have built your strength up to a decent level. Then you'll be able to perform the exercise without any assistance and work on increasing your rep numbers.

You can buy the bands here on Amazon.com: http://www.amazon.com/Green-WODFitters-Resistance-Power-lifting-Christmas/dp/B00IQM3WYK/ref=sr_1_4?s=sports-and-fitness&ie=UTF8&qid=1465199271&sr=1-4&keywords=resistance+bands+pull+up

#8 Pull-ups

A mammoth exercise that blasts the entire upper back, shoulders and arms. Pull-ups also work your core area to an extent as you balance your body during the movement.

Slightly harder than chin-ups, but so effective for developing muscle tone. As you build up your strength you will also naturally increase your reps.

Technique

\>> Grab a pull-up bar with your hands positioned at wider than shoulder width and your palms facing outwards.

\>> Pull your body upwards and cross your legs as soon as they leave the floor.

\>> Pull hard until your shoulers are level with your hands and then lower your body to the starting position.

Common mistakes

Not dropping your body low enough. Again this is only half a rep and simply won't work your muscles hard enough. Your arms should lock out at the bottom.

Swinging your head and body. It's not easy to balance your body during pull-ups, but focus on using the full range of your arms to raise and lower your body, rather than trying to 'nudge' yourself upwards at the top.

Muscles worked: Shoulders, lats, trapezius, forearms, triceps, abs.

#9 Dips

I've heard this one being nicknamed 'The Upper Body Squat' – and no wonder, it is an outstanding exercise that engages most parts of your upper body.

Technique

\>> Grab both handles of the dip bar and straighten your arms, keeping your body rigid and crossing over your legs.

\>> Looking straight ahead, bend your elbows and lower your body in a controlled way until your arms are at a 90 degree angle (i.e. your upper arms are parallel with the floor).

>> Focusing on keeping your body rigid, push your body upwards again until your arms are straight and your elbows lock out.

Common mistakes to avoid

Swinging your body. Balance is important and it's all too easy to swing forward or backwards as you perform this exercise. Keep your body firm and your gaze straight ahead to avoid doing this.

Not dipping low enough. A very common mistake is where people only lower their body slightly, sometimes only a few inches. It's important to hit that 90 degree angle to properly work the muscles.

Muscles worked: shoulders, chest, triceps, forearms, abs.

#10 Military Press

A straightforward but highly effective compound exercise for developing your upper body.

Technique

>> Stand with your legs apart and hold a barbell at just above your upper chest area, with your elbows slightly below a 90 degree angle.

>> Press the bar firmly above your head until your elbows lock out, then lower to the starting position.

Common mistakes to avoid

Swaying backwards or forwards during the exercise. Keep your feet planted in the same position throughout.

Muscles worked: Shoulders, chest, trapezius, triceps, forearms.

Chapter 6

Muscle Isolation Moves

Compounds are king and will form the majority of our workouts, but we'll also include some isolation exercises.

We're sculpting stronger, better bodies here, so think of it like this: compounds are the sculptor's clay for creating the athletic, muscular physique...and isolation exercises are his carving tools for definition.

There are countless variations of isolation exercises – enough to fill a book on their own. But it's pointless going into them all because they'll only make up a smaller part of our workouts.

Instead, I've chosen my top three isolation exercises for each of the main muscle groups and listed them below.

CHEST

Dumbbell press

Similar to bench press, but using a dumbbell in each arm instead to work the pectoral muscles.

<u>Technique</u>

>> Lying flat on a bench, hold two dumbbells at slightly wider than shoulder width, with your palms facing outward .

>> Press dumbbells straight up and inwards till they meet in the middle.

>> Squeeze your chest at the very top of the movement for a second and then lower the dumbbells to the same starting position in a controlled way.

Common mistake to avoid

Bashing the dumbbells together at the top of the movement as this can lead to losing balance and poor form.

Dumbbell flyes

Again involving the bench and dumbbells, but hitting the chest muscles in a different way.

Technique

>> Lying flat on a bench, press two dumbbells straight up in the air with your palms are facing inwards.

>> Slowly bring your arms outwards, as if you were stretching, until your upper arms are roughly parallel with the floor. Your arms should be slightly bent and you should feel the strain across your chest and shoulders.

>> Bring your arms back up in a butterfly motion till the dumbbells reach the starting position again.

>> Squeeze your chest muscles at the very top of the movement, before lowering again.

Common mistake to avoid

Raising your lower back off the bench. Keep your upper and lower back firmly on there.

Dumbbell pullover

This great single dumbbell exercise inflates the ribcage area – and your chest if you give it enough attention!

Technique

>> Lie flat on a bench, with your head in line with the very top of it. Hold a dumbbell straight above your head using your two palms.

>> Keeping your arms straight, slowly lower the dumbbell backwards over your head and towards the floor.

>> Once you feel the full stretch on your ribcage and your arms can't lower any further, raise the dumbbell back to the starting position while keeping your arms straight.

Common mistake to avoid

Bending the arms. Keep them as straight as possible throughout the movement.

SHOULDERS

Arnie press

Named after Mr Schwarzenegger because he introduced this twisting style of exercise to really work the shoulders hard. It's a little tricky to master at first, but you'll soon get comfortable with it.

Technique

>> With a bench set in the upright position your back firmly against it, press two dumbbells straight above your head, with your palms facing outwards.

\>\> Bend your elbows and slowly lower the weights – but gradually twist your palms inwards as you do so.

\>\> In the final third of the movement your palms should be facing inwards and your forearms should come together side by side.

\>\> In a reverse motion, open up your arms again and twist your palms outwards while simultaneously pressing the dumbbells.

\>\> Do this twist/press until the dumbbells meet at the starting position, with your palms facing outwards again.

<u>Common mistake to avoid</u>

Not pulling your arms in far enough at the bottom of the movement. Bring your forearms close in together until they are side by side.

Deltoid raises

Dumbbells called into action again and doing a mix of two lifts to hit the front and medial deltoids (aka shoulder muscles).

<u>Technique</u>

\>\> Stand straight holding two dumbbells by your side.

\>\> With your palms facing inwards, raise the dumbbells up in front of you to shoulder height. Pause for a second and then lower them to the starting position.

\>\> For your next rep, turn your hands inward and then raise your arms directly up from the side until shoulder height. Pause briefly again before lowering the weights to your sides again.

\>> Alternate between the two front and side variations throughout the set until failure.

<u>Common mistake to avoid</u>

Letting your arms just drop back down again. Lower them in a controlled way.

Reverse flyes

Using dumbbells to effectively target the rear shoulder muscles.

<u>Technique</u>

\>> Stand with your feet together and knees slightly bent.

\>> Bend forward holding dumbbells together facing inwards and while looking straight ahead.

\>> Raise your arms out to the side (in the opposite motion to chest dumbbell flyes).

\>> Lift the weights as high as possible – while keeping your back in the same position – and lower again to the start.

<u>Common mistake to avoid</u>

Swinging your back up and down during the exercise. Stay steady and only move your arms.

BACK

Cable row

99.9% of gyms have these machines and they're great for isolating the lats, helping develop an athletic v-shaped back.

Technique

>> Place your feet on the foot-rests and your shins/knees against the pads, effectively locking your legs in position.

>> Grab the cable handle and sit up straight, keeping your back rigid.

>> Pull the cable handle towards you until it almost touches your lower chest.

>> Slowly release the handle and cable back to its starting position.

Common mistake to avoid

Moving your back forwards and backwards. Keeps your hips and back in the same upright position throughout the move.

Lat pulldown

This is like a machine variation of the pull-up...but not nearly as effective as that compound exercise.

Technique

>> The bench may have pads you can rest your knees under, which helps hold your body in position. If it does, then use them.

>> ...but first grab the bar from above your head, with your hands in a position slightly wider than your shoulders.

>> Pull the bar down as close to your upper chest as feels comfortable.

>> Return the bar and cable back to its starting position in a controlled way.

Common mistake to avoid

Raising your lower body off the bench as you return the weight to the starting position. Keep your legs and waist in place, locking them in position under the pads if the machine has them.

Dumbbell row

Another great exercise for targeting the lats and therefore hitting a large portion of your back.

Technique

>> Rest your right knee/shin and your straight right arm on a bench, holding yourself in position.

>> Keep your left leg straight at the side and grab a dumbbell from the floor with your left arm.

>> Pull the dumbbell towards your body until your arm is at a 90 degree angle.

>> Lower your weight back to the starting position until your arm is straight again.

>> Do a full set and then switch round, placing your left limbs on the bench, so you can then work your right side.

Common mistake to avoid

Moving your shoulder up and down. Focus on keeping the arm resting on the bench completely straight throughout as this will hold your body in position.

BICEPS

Barbell curls

The standard biceps exercise that everyone recognises. Great move for isolating the biceps and also hitting the forearms.

Technique

>> Stand with your back straight and hold a barbell at your thighs, with an underhand grip and your arms at shoulder width.

>> Keeping your elbows tucked in against your waist, curl the bar upwards towards your chest.

>> Squeeze your biceps at the top for a second and then lower the bar in a controlled way down to your thighs again.

Common mistake to avoid

Swinging your body to gain momentum and help lift the bar. Focus on keeping your body rigid throughout the movement, with your upper arms flat against your body and your elbows locked in position at your waist. Only your forearms should be moving up and down like a lever.

Lying bench curls

Curling with dumbbells this time and by lying at an angle you put additional strain on the biceps. Exactly what we want!

Technique

>> Set a bench to a slight incline, but not too high or too low (see picture for ideal level).

\>\> Lie back on the bench with a dumbbell in each hand and start with your arms completely straight down each side.

\>\> Fix your gaze on something directly above you to stay focused.

\>\> While keeping your upper arms and elbows in the same position, curls the dumbbells up close to your shoulders.

\>\> Squeeze your biceps as you hold the dumbbells at the top for a second – and then slowly lower to the starting position.

Common mistake to avoid

Raising your waist or back off the bench. Keep your body firmly placed against the bench and move only from the elbows.

21's

This is basically barbell curls again – but with a bicep burning twist. It involves 21 continuous reps and is a great move to include near the end of your workout as it is really effective for reaching muscle fatigue.

Technique

\>\> Get in the same starting position as you would with the barbell curl – but decrease the weight by ¼ or 1/3 because you will be completing more reps at once.

\>\> With your upper arms firmly against your side and working only from the elbow again, curl the bar upwards. However, only come halfway up this time – until your forearms are parallel with the floor – and then lower the weight to your thighs once more.

\>\> Do this for 7 reps.

\>\> Then hold the bar with your arms bent at a 90 degree angle and curl up to your chest – like you would in only the second part of a normal bicep curl.

\>\> Lower the bar, but only till the halfway point where your arms reach that 90 degree angle again.

\>\> Do this for another 7 reps.

\>\> Without pausing for a rest, then move straight into full barbell curls, lifting from your thighs all the way up to your chest.

\>\> Do this for a final 7 reps until you have completed 21 in total.

<u>Common mistake to avoid</u>

Lifting the barbell too high in the first part, or lowering it too low in the second part of 21's. Remember to only go halfway each time, which makes the arms work hard to control the weight – and then makes the final 7 reps much tougher.

TRICEPS

Narrow press

This move is basically bench pressing, but with a narrow grip which brings the tricep muscles into action.

<u>Technique</u>

\>\> Set up a barbell and bench as you would for bench pressing, but <u>decrease the weight by at least 1/3</u> as the narrow grip makes this a bit more tricky to balance the bar.

\>\> Grab the bar and move your hands inwards by a couple of inches, so that they are narrower than shoulder width.

\>\> Lift the bar off the catches and straighten your arms till you're holding it comfortably and feel balanced.

\>\> Then lower the bar to the middle part of your chest and press back to the top until your elbows lock out.

Common mistake to avoid

The bar swaying from side to side. It's a bit awkward to balance at first because of the narrow grip but focus on holding the bar steady at the start before beginning your reps.

Cable pushdown

Is a cable machine exercise, this involves pushing a bar downwards rather than pressing or pulling it to engage the triceps muscles.

Technique

\>\> Set the pin in the machine to a suitable weight level.

\>\> Set the cable pulley to the top of the machine and attach either a straight bar, or ideally one with a bend that allows your hands to slope downwards.

\>\> Stand up straight with your feet apart and grab the bar with an overhand grip. Then pull the bar down to your thighs until your arms are straight.

\>\> Keeping your back straight and upper arms tucked against your side, raise the bar until your forearms are slightly higher than being parallel to the floor.

\>\> Push the bar back down to your thighs until your arms lock out.

Common mistake to avoid

Swinging the bar upwards and raising your arms too high. This can be avoided by focusing on keeping your upper arms pressed against your side and your elbows in the same spot throughout.

Overhead rope extension

Another cable machine exercise, but this time involving pressing a rope outwards. Can be a bit tricky to master at first, so start with a light weight until confident with the move.

Technique

\>> Set the cable pulley to the top of the machine and attach a short rope.

\>> Facing outwards away from the machine, grab the rope from behind your head with your fists.

\>> Step forward and bend your kness, while your elbows are raised next to your head as you pull the rope forward.

\>> This is the position to hold your body in throughout – as the only part of your body to move is your forearms.

\>> Holding the rope tight, press it forward past your head until your arms are straight in front of you. (Feel free to whip out a cape and pretend you're Superman).

\>> While keeping your elbows in position at the side of your head, bring your fists backwards again behind your head.

Common mistake to avoid

Not bending forward enough at the beginning. Bend your knees and lean forward from the waist to get in the correct starting position.

LEGS

Quad machine

Seated leg curl machine that totally isolates the quadriceps muscles.

<u>Technique</u>

>> Adjust the levers on the machine so that your back is well supported and the cushioned bar is resting back against your lower shin, effectively locking your legs in position.

>> Hold the bars at either side of the machine and curl your legs upwards until your calves are parallel with the floor and you can feel the tension on your thighs.

>> Lower the weight to the starting position in a controlled manner.

<u>Common mistake to avoid</u>

Arching your back. This is a shortcut to injury so keep your back firmly pressed against the rest behind you. Holding the bars at the side of the machine also help keep you in place.

Hamstring machine

Virtually the reverse of the quad machine, curling from the top downwards and isolating the hamstring muscles.

<u>Technique</u>

>> Sit on the chair with your legs straight, resting your heels on the cushioned bar that is furthest away.

>> Make sure your back is supported and then pull the other cushioned bar on to your lower thighs and lock it in position.

\>\> Push downwards with your heels, curling the bar inwards until the soles of your feet are virtually parallel with the floor.

\>\> Hold for a second and then raise your legs to the top again in a controlled way.

<u>Common mistake to avoid</u>

Not bringing the bar down low enough. Ensure you curl your legs in until the soles of your shoes are facing the floor.

Dumbbell lunges

One step forward, bending the knees, with a dumbbell in each hand. Really effective move for toning the glutes too.

<u>Technique</u>

\>\> Stand up straight with your arms by your side, holding a dumbbell in each hand.

\>\> Take a step forward, bending your legs as if you're about to propose to some unlucky person.

\>\> Keeping your shoulders and back straight, lower your body until your trailing knee almost touches the floor. Push back into the starting position and then repeat with the other leg.

<u>Common mistake to avoid</u>

Rounding your shoulders, or leaning forward too far, which can put you off balance. Keep your upper body rigid and your arms straight down by your sides.

EXERCISE TIPS

\>\> Try to perform them all in front of a mirror. This is the best way to maintain proper technique.

\>\> In the eccentric (second part of every exercise) always make sure you lower the weight in a controlled way. You'll work the muscles harder – and be less likely to get injured.

\>\> Never drop or smash your weights off the floor. It ain't cool. Only Meatheads do that.

Chapter 7

How To Create Your Own Training Plans

I've had to learn all sorts of new things over the past couple of years just to get this book in your hands. I've been writing for a wee while but...getting the book on Kindle? Creating a paperback version? Building my fitness business website?

I didn't have a clue what I was doing. I could have spent 23.5 years trying to figure it all out...or I could have paid an expert to lead the way and save me light years.

Same applies to strength training, a healthy diet and your body transformation. A personal training and nutrition coach with plenty of experience can give you a shortcut to success.

For beginners, I'd always recommend signing up to a proven programme with a personal trainer as the accountability alone can be invaluable. But for those who want to go it alone, this chapter will equip you with a simple method for designing your own workouts.

We already have the exercises. We already have a solid guide for reps and sets. Now we'll introduce effective training systems.

This chapter will also provide sound advice on training intensity and rest periods to avoid possible burnout.

Let's get started...

Variety + Progressive Overload = Progress

The two main components of an effective weight training routine are *progressive overload* and *variety*. If every gym day feels like Groundhog Day then obviously you won't stick at it long.

Variety is not just essential for keeping you motivated and making good progress, it'll also consistently challenge you and add an element of excitement to each workout.

It's easy to chop and change by mixing up countless variations of compound and isolation exercises, the order you complete them in, and varying your rest time.

Through *progressive overload* we gradually increase the weight resistance on our muscles.

The aim should always be to go as heavy as possible - whether you're a male, female or filthy animal – but without letting your technique slip. (Remember, if you can't manage 6 reps then you're going too heavy, if you can manage more than 9 then it's time to up the weight).

The science behind progressive overload is that the added resistance induces muscle hypertrophy, which leads to growth and development. Instead of performing 3 sets of 10 reps of with the *same* weight for weeks and months at a time, you add more weight as the body strengthens and adapts

Your muscles get wise to doing the same routine with the same weight. This does nothing for the development of your physique and will leave your body looking flat. By increasing the weight in stages you are continually causing tears in the muscle fibres, prompting a repair, growth and adapting cycle.

How To Design Your Own Workout Plan

Step #1

Select 7-8 exercises from the previous two chapters – but make the majority of them compounds. (i.e. *Squats, deadlifts, chin-ups, upright row, bent over row, military press*...and *lunges* and *cable row* as your isolation moves).

Step #2

Apply the 3,6,9 Principle (3 sets and aiming for between 6 and 9 reps each time) for these exercises. This is ideal for achieving muscle fatigue and progressive overload as it indicates when you're ready to increase your weights, or decrease them if need be.

Step #3

Choose a training system to combine all of the above. There are many different training approaches, and they all have their pros and cons. Below I've listed what I consider to be the most effective.

<u>Select one of them and use it for 4-6 weeks before switching to another.</u>

This ensures the body doesn't adapt to any particular routine and keeps shocking the muscles – which helps stimulate more growth and development.

Four Top Training Systems

Three Set Shocker

For each exercise complete two sets of a heavy weight, focusing on proper technique for every rep. Have up to 90 seconds rest between these sets.

Then immediately after completing the second set <u>lower the weight by one third</u> and jump straight into a third 'shocker' set.

By giving your muscles little or no rest after their 90 second breather first time around we're aiming to shock them into shape.

Workout example (all listed kilogram weights are random examples, find your own suitable weight using the 3,6,9 Principle):

- Squats 90kg >> 90 secs rest >> squats 90kg >> 0-20 secs rest >> squats 60kg.

- Clean and press 45kg >> 90 secs rest >>clean and press 45kg >> 0-20 secs rest >> clean and press 30kg.

- Lunges 50kg >> 90 secs rest >> Dumbbell lunges 50kg >> 0-20 secs rest >> dumbbell lunges 35kg.

- Bent over row 65kg >> 90 secs rest >> bent over row 65kg >> 0-20 secs rest >> bent over row 45kg.

- Pull-ups max amount of reps >> 90 secs rest >> Pull-ups max amount of reps >>0-20 secs rest >>pull-ups max mount of reps.

- Military press 45kg >> 90 secs rest >> military press 45kg >> 0-20 secs rest >> military press 30kg.

- Barbell curls 30kg >> 90 secs rest >> barbell curls 30kg >> 0-20 secs rest >> barbell curls 20kg.

The Slow Burner

For each exercise do two sets as heavy as you can go...remember to aim for between 6 and 9 reps. Allow for up to 90 seconds rest after your first and second set.

Then drop the weight by half and complete a final set – but with a slightly different approach.

Begin each exercise normally and then squeeze the muscles when they are contracting at the peak of the exercise. Then lower the weight more slowly in the eccentric part of the movement.

For example: when bench pressing lower the bar slowly for 2-3 seconds. When it reaches your chest hold it for 2 secs before pushing firmly back to the top. Then repeat.

Another example: when doing bicep curls, raise the bar as you normally would. But as you reach the top of the movement hold and squeeze your biceps for 2 secs. Then slowly lower the bar downwards for 2-3 secs. Then repeat.

Workout example (5 compounds, 3 isolation exercises):

- Deadlifts 80kg >> 90 secs rest >> deadlifts 80kg >> 90 secs rest >> deadlifts 40kg slow reps.
- Bench press 70kg >> 90 secs rest >> bench press 70kg >> 90 secs rest >> bench press 35kg slow.
- Clean and press 45kg >> 90 secs rest >> clean and press 45kg >> 90 secs rest >> clean and press 22.5kg or 25kg slow reps.
- Chin-ups >> 90 secs rest >> chin-ups >> 90 secs rest >> slow chin-ups.

- Upright row 40kg >> 90 secs rest >> upright row 40kg >> 90 secs rest >> upright row 20kg slow.

- Dumbbell flyes 25kg >> 90 secs rest >> Dumbbell flyes 25kg >> 90 secs rest >> Dumbbell flyes 12.5kg

- Dips >> 90 secs rest >> dips >> 90 secs rest >> slow dips.

- Triceps bar pushdown 55kg >> 90 secs rest >> triceps bar pushdown 55kg >> 90 secs rest >> slow triceps bar pushdown 27kg or 30kg

Drop Sets

This system involves starting with a weight where you can manage 6-9 reps, followed by two consecutive sets where you drop the load by about 20%-25% each time.

For example, a barbell row may start at 60kg, the second set would drop to 45kg, and third set would be done at around 35kg. Sounds easy enough, right?

Not really, because you are only allowed up to 30 seconds rest between each set. The weight may be decreasing each time, but the shorter recovery period ensures it doesn't feel like it.

The drop sets system is much easier with a training partner because they can unload the bar between sets while you catch your breath.

Workout example (6 compounds, 2 isolation exercises):

- Bench press 70kg >> 30 secs rest max >> Bench press 55kg >> 30 secs rest max >> bench press 45kg.

- Dumbbell flyes 25kg >> 30 secs rest max >> dumbbell flyes 20kg >> 30 secs rest max >> dumbbell flyes 15kg.

- Deadlifts 80kg >> 30 secs rest >> deadlifts 60kg >> 30 secs rest >> deadlifts 50kg.

- Chin-ups >> 30 secs rest max >> chin-ups >> 30 secs rest max >> chin-ups.

- Military press 50kg >> 30 secs rest max >> military press 35kg >> 30 secs rest max >> military press 25kg.

- Bent over row 65kg >> 30 secs rest max >> bent over row 50kg >> 30 secs rest max >> bent over row 40kg.

- Lat pulldown 70kg >> 30 secs rest max >> lat pulldown 55kg >> 30 secs rest max >> lat pulldown 45kg.

- Lying bench curls 12.5kg >> 30 secs rest max >> lying bench curls 10kg >> 30 secs rest max >> 7.5kg.

The 25's

Still three sets. Still lifting heavy. Only difference is you're aiming to complete a combined total of at least 25 reps.

If you exceed 25 mark a '+' in your training diary to step it up a level next time.

The difficulty with this system is that by the third set your muscles will be tiring, but you're maintaining the same heavy weight (unlike drop sets or the three sets shocker).

The upside is that you should give yourself up to 90 secs rest in between every set to prepare. Also, you're less concerned with the number of reps in an individual set than you are with the sum total.

For example, if you only manage 8 reps in your first two sets of biceps curls you know that it's not impossible to still achieve a '+' by really going for it in the final set.

That is when it is time to get some good music on, turn it up loud, and stay focused on the number 9 in your head. On the other hand, this system is particularly good for bodyweight exercises such as press ups, dips, pull-ups and chin-ups. By the third set you will likely be knackered and manage maybe only 5 or 6 – but if you racked up 11 and 8, or 10 and 9, in your first two sets then you can still hit 25 in total.

If you're a complete beginner then a resistance band is highly recommended. No matter how many reps you get, mark it in your training diary and just keep aiming to outdo yourself.

Workout example (5 compounds, 2 isolation exercises)

- Squats 80kg >> 90 secs rest >> Squats 80kg >> 90 secs rest >> Squats 80kg.

- Incline bench press 60kg >> 90 secs rest >> incline bench press 60kg >> 90 secs rest >> incline bench press.

- Cable machine row 60kg >> 90 secs rest >> cable machine row 60kg >> 90 secs rest >> cable machine row 60kg.

- Clean and press 50kg >> 90 secs rest >> clean and press 50kg >> 90 secs rest >> clean and press 50kg.

- Chin-ups >> 90 secs rest >> chin-ups >> 90 secs rest >> chin-ups.

- Upright row 45kg >> 90 secs rest >> upright row 45kg >> 90 secs rest >> upright row 45kg.

- Dumbbell flyes 15kg >> 90 secs rest >> dumbbell flyes 15kg >> 90 secs rest >> dumbbell flyes 15kg.

You Call The Shots…Give Your All With Every Rep

These are all just workout examples, none of it is set in stone. It's simply to demonstrate how you can create an endless variety of weight training workouts.

You choose the exercises.

You choose the order you want to do them in.

You select the weight that's right for you.

I'd always recommend doing at least 7 exercises – <u>and ensuring that compounds make up the majority of your workout</u>. (Have I mentioned how important compounds are yet??) Whether that's at a 6:2 ratio with isolation exercises, a 5:3 or 7:1 ratio…or even just all compounds.

You may even want to expand your workout to do 9 or 10 exercises. That's cool, but it's not necessary to go beyond that when you train this way. Stick to the advice in this chapter – and just give your all with every single rep!

CHECKLIST

- Variety and progressive overload are key to making good progress in building muscle and burning fat.

- To keep things fresh you simply mix up countless variations of compound and isolation exercises, the order you complete them in, and by utilising different training systems.

- Through progressive overload we always aim to increase the weight - but not at the expense of proper technique.

- Progressive overload induces hypertrophy, which leads to muscle growth and development.

- Design your own workout plan in three simple steps.

1 – Select 7 or 8 exercises, the majority of which should be compounds.

2 – Apply the 3,6,9 Principle for reps and sets.

3 – Choose a training system.

- There are four recommended training systems: Three Set Shocker; Slow Burner; Drop Sets; and 25's.

- Apply one training system for 4-6 weeks and then switch to another to keep shocking the muscles.

- Stay consistent. Then the muscle will come...and the fat will go.

Chapter 8

9 Essential Ingredients To Better Nutrition

Following the right diet is a bit like politics: most people have an opinion on it...and no-one is ever right.

The Paleo crowd will tell you that we should eating like cavemen, vegans will argue that you shouldn't touch meat, and following the alkaline diet means you'll live until you're 193 apparently...

I'll be honest, I've tried all of the above – and plenty other diets. This was simply down to having a dodgy stomach in my 20's and I wanted to figure out what foods were easiest on my messed-up digestive system.

What I found from nearly a decade of experimentation is that each diet has its upsides and downsides. Each diet has similarities. And most of them share a few core principles (i.e. everyone agrees that refined sugar is bad for you and too much makes you fat).

But I don't even like the word 'diet', it makes me think of something we're chained to and need to struggle through. Fact is, we need food to survive...and stuffing our faces is one of the best things about being alive!

I'll never give up Chinese takeaway food as long as I live...I love chicken and ham fried rice (with prawn crackers) wayyy too much. I'll carry on having a cappuccino when I want one, and I'll eat some chocolate occasionally.

Here's what I tell my online personal training clients: **eat as clean as possible Monday-Friday and then cut loose a bit at the weekend.**

By 'cut loose' I obviously don't mean have a KFC chicken bucket for breakfast on Saturday followed a pizza and half a tub of ice cream for dinner. But by allowing yourself the odd treat at the weekend and not being as strict with your food, you're much more likely to stick with healthy eating throughout the rest of the week.

And when you're training properly in the gym three days per week as described in this book, you'll eventually raise your metabolism to a level where you'll be a fat burning machine anyway! But what exactly does eating 'clean' most of the week involve?

#1 Avoid alcohol

Not simply because the booze is bad for you, but because of how much garbage we eat afterwards. Hangovers lower our blood sugar, make us feel terrible...and what do we do to feel better?

Eat mountains of junk food. Hungover people naturally crave sugar, fat and simple carbs as a quick way to raise their blood sugar levels.

Now I'm in my thirties, hangovers don't just hang around on a Sunday...I'm still feeling it by Tuesday morning!

#2 Reduce sugar intake

If you're exercising regularly but still eating a diet high in sugar then you're wasting your time. Fats have got a bad rap for years, but the real enemy to fantastic health and a great physique is the sweet stuff.

The liver can only store so much glycogen from sugars and when there's too much sugar in the diet, this glycogen is converted to fatty acids and released back into the body. This is then stored as bodyfat in areas you don't want...belly, chest, arms, ass.

My number one piece of dietary advice for anyone looking to improve their physique, whether their priority is losing weight or adding muscle mass, is to reduce sugar intake as much as possible.

Health experts recommend that we only have around 25g-30g (6 teaspoons) of added sugar per day. There are 35g of sugar in a small can of Coke!

Go for one sugar instead of two in tea or coffee, or even better, swap these drinks for herbal teas or water. Stop eating desserts after dinner, ditch fizzy drinks, eat something like scrambled eggs with wholemeal bread rather than cereals, which are often high in sugar.

#3 Cook fresh

Stock up on fresh foods, plenty of vegetables etc, and cook meals at home from scratch rather than popping a ready meal in the microwave. Firstly, you know exactly what ingredients are going into your meal and there won't be any dodgy additives or preservatives in there.

Secondly, the microwave zaps the life out of your food, meaning there's very little left in the way of vitamins and minerals by the time you hear that 'ding' noise.

Not a good cook? Neither was I. There are tons of good cook books out there and some of the recipes are outrageously good. I'd highly recommend Jamie Oliver's 30 Minute Meals from Amazon. An even easier option for recipes....Google.

#4 Cook double the amount of food for dinner

Then take it into work for lunch the next day. This is an easy healthy habit to get into.

Cooking freshly-made healthy dinners regularly at home is the way forward for eating clean – and you can kill two birds with one stone by cooking plenty and munching on the rest for lunch the next day.

It means you won't buy fast food or an unhealthy option from the work canteen.

#5 Don't buy in junk food

If there are chocolate, biscuits, potato chips etc in your cupboards within easy reach then they're going to get devoured at some point. Just remove the tempting foods completely by bodyswerving them at the supermarket.

Buy in plenty of vegetables and fruit, and stock up on healthy snacks such as packets of nuts and raisins, hummus, and oatcakes and natural unsweetened peanut butter (my favourite snack which is really filling).

#6 Refrain from hitting that 'snooze' button 23 times

If you regularly get out of bed late and rush around in the morning your diet will always suffer. It's hard eating clean when you've only got 30 minutes to get showered, dressed, brush your teeth, get to work…and then think about filling your belly.

Set the alarm a bit earlier than normal, keep your filthy paws away from that snooze button, make yourself a delicious dish, and eat it in a civilised, non-manic manner.

Which takes us on to the next tip…

#7 Get breakfast ready the night before

Want a foolproof way of getting your day off to a healthy, clean eating start? (Like, if you don't trust yourself not to hit the snooze button constantly).

Make a healthy breakfast shake the night before. Just Google 'healthy smoothie recipes' or 'clean eating smoothie' to get plenty of shake ideas. You can then grab the shaker as you run out the door and drink that one the way to work, rather than swinging past a fast food drive thru for a greasy breakfast.

#8 Think about how crappy you'll feel *afterwards*

The treats, sweets, and fast food are hard to resist sometimes because they taste so good. That's usually what's on our minds when we get stuck into the less than healthy food.

But how do you usually feel <u>after</u> a splurge when you've been trying to eat clean? The guilt usually kicks in pretty sharpish, doesn't it? And there's a fair chance you'll feel bloated, tired, maybe even a bit sick after a large fast food meal.

When you're struggling with the temptation of junk food, first focus on this familiar not-so-good feeling that usually occurs after you go off the rails. It takes a bit of practice and perseverance but it can help you stay on track.

#9 Cut yourself a bit of slack at the weekend

Making the right food choices consistently is hugely important, but don't treat eating and nutrition like some sort of military exercise. It'll never work – as most fad diets prove in the long run.

You'll only end up miserable and back at square one. Going round in circles.

As I mentioned earlier in this chapter, why not focus on eating super clean Monday-Friday, and then cut yourself a bit of slack at the weekend?

Enjoy your favourite takeaway meal on a Saturday night with some wine. Or popcorn and some chocolate while watching a movie.

As long as you don't go overboard, you'll still be able to make progress in your health and fitness goals.

Knowing the rules are relaxed a bit at the weekend makes it much more likely you'll stick with the clean eating masterplan for the majority of the week.

CHECKLIST

- Avoid the big bad booze as much as you can. It'll only make you feel like crap and then the low blood sugar levels will have you eating more junk food in one day than you would in a week!

- Eat as clean as possible Monday-Friday and then cut loose a little at the weekend.

- Reduce sugar intake as much as possible because excess sugar is stored as body fat.

- Cook fresh regularly and avoid fast food/ready meals as much as you can.

- Making large amounts of food for dinner and then taking a serving into work for lunch the next day is a good healthy habit to get into.

- Try not to keep hitting the snooze button repeatedly. You'll likely get up late, not have time to prepare proper healthy food for breakfast and lunch, and will grab some convenience junk food.

- A healthy shake can be made in minutes the night before, and you can grab this in the morning for breakfast or lunch.

- Step away from the cakes...simply don't buy in junk food. Clear away temptation by replacing the crappy foods with healthier snacks such as nuts and raisins, fruit etc.

Chapter 9

10 Reasons You've Not Been Building Muscle And Losing Fat

What if you've been exercising hard for years? What if you've always been a healthy eater? What if you seem to be doing things right...but the muscle just ain't coming and/or the flab just ain't shifting?

It can be head-explodingly frustrating when there's not much to show for all the hours of gym work. Especially when you've got some freak of nature pals like me who put in less effort, eat more junk and yet they still manage to stay in good shape.

I've pulled together my top 11 reasons for a lack of success in building muscle and losing fat. Some of them touch upon areas already covered in the book – but underline the importance of avoiding commonly made mistakes.

This puts you in a position where you can see where you've maybe gone wrong in the past. You'll also know exactly what needs adjusting to get real results.

I've made every single one of these mistakes myself in the past, and I'll still occasionally slip-up with two or three them. Stuff happens in life that can throw our training, diet and healthy lifestyle out of whack.

This often results in one or more of the 11 consequences listed in this chapter. The important thing is simply to get back on track as quickly as you can. When I look back to my life about 10 years ago I was constantly making three of these mistakes – and it affected both my weight training results and health.

I was hitting the gym four times per week and eating a clean diet. I was lifting heavy, doing squats, deadlifts, all the big movements I rave about these days. My nutrition was good: good sources of protein, fruit and veg, and very little junk food. Doing everything right on those two major fronts.

But I *still* wasn't seeing any noticeable results in muscle size or definition. I've always been a 'hard gainer' – aka skinny dude who struggles to get bigger – but it seemed like I just couldn't add one single pound of muscle. It was doing my head in.

At that time, I was struggling with my old job at the time and was pretty highly-strung and feeling anxious Monday-Friday.

The only time I really chilled out was at the weekend when I wasn't in the office. This led to an unhealthy cycle of feeling zapped of energy after work, going to the gym partly to try and relieve the stress...but then not recovering properly from my workouts because I was only getting 4-5 hours of sleep per night.

Stress and lack of sleep are a bad combination – and you'll see why they're a block to a brilliant body in reasons 7 and 9.

Back then I was also playing football (badly) with my mates one, sometimes two, nights per week in addition to my gym training sessions. As a slim guy with a pretty high metabolism, these high energy games were eating into my muscle gains.

The odd 20-30 minute session of intense cardio – such as sprints or circuit training – is really good for conditioning. My problem was that I was doing 60-120 minutes of it per week and expending too many calories. As a result, my body also used some of my protein stores for fuel and I lost muscle gains.

My health is more important than work, and muscle is way more important than football. So I ditched the football and finally cut back on the extra hours in the office. I also found the answer to both the stress and sleep problems – magnesium oil and meditation.

10 Blocks To Building Muscle And Burning Fat Effectively

#1 Wasting your time on cardio

Cardio is crap. Simple as that. Jogging, running, aerobics, fitness classes may well burn calories – but they do zilch for adding muscle mass or developing the proper definition you're looking for.

These forms of standard cardio are also less effective at stripping away fat anyway. While both cardio and weight training elevate your metabolism levels, the post-workout burn continues for much longer periods with weight training.

Studies have shown that metabolic rates can stay heightened for more than 24 hours afterwards. Your body effectively turns into a muscle building, fat burning machine...while you sleep. Result!

#2 Not continually raising the bar

Two words to always keep in mind when weight training: go heavy. Doesn't matter whether you're a man, woman, young or old, the way to initiate real change in the shape and strength of your body is to properly test it with serious resistance.

This is obviously pointless without proper technique - no swinging, swaying or half reps - as strict form is crucial to working the muscle correctly.

You will develop strength quicker than you think. You will often be able to do more reps than before. You will start lifting heavier than you thought you could.

It's up to you to keep pushing on so that the body doesn't adapt. Not only is this gym work about pressing and pulling the bar, it's about continually raising it too.

#3 Focusing on the wrong weightlifting exercises

This means skipping the biggest and best moves – compound exercises. Yes I do sound like a badly broken record, but the squats, deadlifts, bench press, chin-ups etc have got to be at the forefront of your training.

These are the most effective exercises for building muscle, stoking up the fat burning fire, and optimal body composition. Yet I'd guess that less than half of people I see lifting weights in the gym include these moves.

Why? Because they're tough, especially when you're lifting heavy. But the easy route leads nowhere good. Let the rest of them take that path while you charge along the road to real results.

#4 Eating junk food

Eating healthy, natural, unprocessed, freshly cooked food the majority of the time is the way forward. It should never feel like you're on a diet, and it doesn't mean you have to give up the odd treat.

At the same time, you've got to realise that <u>too much</u> junk food will hamper your efforts. While this type of weight training will add muscle and torch fat extremely effectively, a diet with excess sugar and highly processed foods simply leads to more fat being stored again.

#5 Messing up your calorie intake

Calories from our foods are used by the body for energy. Regularly take in more than you expend and you'll gain weight...and vice versa.

A slim guy like me is never going to add another pound of muscle if I regularly fall below the extra calories my body needs for tough training sessions. For someone who is overweight, their body will not use up their fat stores for energy if they continue taking in an excessive amount of calories every day.

I'd never recommend you keep a constant count of calories, life's too short. But you should at least have a fair idea of how many are in the foods you're eating and your personal requirements based on your health and fitness goals.

#6 Not drinking enough water

The body is made up of around 65% water and us humans generally agree we'd be pretty screwed without it.

But plenty of water is also very important for muscle strength and size, particularly when supplementing with creatine as this pulls more fluid into the muscles. Studies have also shown that just a small drop in water of 4% can cause a loss of muscular strength and endurance. In order to stay strong you must stay hydrated.

The European Food Safety Authority recommends around 2.5 litres per day for men and 2 litres per day for women, while the USDA (United States Department For Agriculture) tells us adult men and women should be drinking 2.7 litres daily.

The numbers vary with different health authorities, but taking into account sweating during training, men and women lifting weights should shoot closer to 3 litres per day.

#7 Not getting enough sleep

Don't underestimate how detrimental a lack of sleep can be. The hard work may be done in the gym, but muscle is built in bed. Your sleeping hours are when the body develops. It sets to work repairing the tears caused to muscle fibres during weight training.

This is supported by the release of anabolic hormones including testosterone and growth hormone during your sleep. Medical experts say the body releases testosterone between 2am and 6am, so it's wise not to interrupt this process through staying up late or broken sleep patterns.

Minimum seven hours, but eight is even better. Late night TV, texting on your mobile phone, or messing around on Facebook not long before you go to bed all keep the brain stimulated – and make it difficult to nod off. Getting into a routine where you generally go to bed and get up at the same time will also create a healthy pattern where you're not trying to catch up on lost sleep.

#8 Digestion issues

This is another big factor, yet not properly appreciated. Most people are more concerned about cramming in protein, protein and more protein in the hope of building more muscle...without properly taking digestion into account.

You could eat as much protein as you like, or the best food sources, but you may not be able to *absorb* it properly due to poor gut health. The body gives us warning signs, like a bloated stomach, heartburn or embarrassingly stinky gas, when we're struggling to break down our food.

Stress is a culprit because the digestive system effectively shuts down when we're struggling mentally or emotionally. Eating processed junk over a long period of time also plays its part, and both can negatively affect the ratio of good to bad bacteria in your stomach (which is crucial for digestion).

What's the answer? Introducing digestive enzyme supplements and fermented foods into your diet can help you break down your food properly.

#9 Too much stress

Chronic stress can lead to high blood pressure, mineral deficiencies and your overall health taking a nosedive. But it can also sabotage your efforts to gain muscle.

In times of stress your body goes into 'fight or flight' mode and releases the stress hormones adrenaline and cortisol, as it should. Problem is, chronically high levels of cortisol breaks down muscle tissue and can impact the immune system, leaving you feeling run-down.

A second knock-on effect of high stress levels is that it can affect your sleep. In times of stress, anxiety, or worry the brain struggles to shut down properly. This can lead to insomnia – and we've already covered how lack of sleep can affect muscle growth and your body's development.

Do whatever you can to minimise stress. Meditation, a relaxing bath, going for a walk with the dog, whatever you enjoy doing.

#10 Not being consistent

This might be the most important mistake not to make. And just to warn you – I bang on about consistency again in this book's conclusion too. Consistency paired with patience = guaranteed success.

Too often one – or both – of these elements are missing when people set about transforming their physique.

Throwing themselves into a new training regime, all guns blazing at the start with a gym membership, new training clothes, stocking up the fridge with healthy foods.

When the muscle doesn't magically appear within a fortnight they lose interest, begin skipping workouts, and become more magnetically drawn to the McDonald's drive-thru. Five Quarter Pounders, three strawberry milkshakes and one Unhappy Meal later and it's back to square one.

There isn't some 'gain muscle, lose fat quick' masterplan that someone has been hiding from us all this time. Body transformations simply don't happen overnight.

But they DO happen. **You absolutely can become a stronger, healthier, barely recognisable version of you if you...**

- Hit the gym 3-4 days per week – and go heavy.

- Precisely plan your training sessions – and stay accountable to your Gym Bible (aka training diary).

- Keep progressively overloading your muscles – and always mix up your training.

- Become obsessed with outdoing yourself – and aim for personal bests in every workout.

- Supply your body with everything it needs for fuel, growth and recovery through a healthy, whole foods diet.

- Treat your body well by minimising the amount of junk that passes your lips.

- Stay focused on the end game.

...and you do all of the above <u>consistently</u>.

CHECKLIST

- Cardio only serves to burn calories, it does nothing for muscle growth and definition.

- Weight training burns fat more effectively because the post-workout burn lasts much longer.

- Keep raising the bar and keep two words in mind: 'go heavy'.

- Focus primarily on compound exercises, no matter what the majority of others are doing.

- Excess sugar and eating highly processed foods will lead to more fat being stored by the body.

- Calorie intake is important for both muscle gain and fat loss – the MyFitnessPal app will help big time.

- Aim to drink around 3 litres of water per day.

- Sleep for a minimum seven hours, eight is better.

- ...if you can't sleep try magnesium oil. It's insanely good for a deep, restful sleep.

- Do whatever you can to minimise stress. Meditation, a relaxing bath, going for a walk with the dog, whatever you enjoy.

- Stay consistent and patient because it will lead to guaranteed success.

Conclusion

"It's easy to become healthy, fit and vibrant. Easy to become financially independent. It's easy to have a happy family and friendships. It's just a matter of mastering the mundane – of <u>repeating simple little disciplines – done consistently over time</u>, that add up to the biggest accomplishments." – Jeff Olson.

This is a quote from one of my favourite books, The Slight Edge. It's a best-seller that's crammed with wisdom from a guy who has experienced both massive success and huge failures in life.

But I'll pick out one of the key lessons from the book and explain why it's relevant to your health and fitness goals.

Jeff Olson tells us that success is something you experience, gradually, over time by consistently showing up and doing what's necessary.

But failure is just as gradual, by letting seemingly small things slip, and not being patient enough for results to come.

Sure, skipping a gym session won't kill you. Not filling in your training diary won't hurt. Boozing every weekend ain't the end of the world.

But if you want to keep growing, moving forward, improving, getting stronger and leaner…instead of slowing, slipping, sliding backwards…then you have to cut out the crap and stay focused on repeating the simple positive disciplines consistently.

Then you'll be on the right side of the 'Slight Edge' – and also on the right path to real results.

Strength Training Program 101 was written to help people frustrated with their lack of success in transforming their physique. It was also written to empower you to take charge of creating your workout programs, make solid progress in the gym, and ultimately get hooked on strength training.

But my main aim was to simplify weight training, diet and motivation methods so that it's all easier to understand – <u>and easier to maintain</u>. Meatheads are making the uncomplicated way too complicated, and that's why so many folk quit too early. Convoluted training regimes and crazy regimented diets.

Who wants to live like that every day? How long can it really last? And where's the fun in it? Transforming your body, and improving your health, through weight training and a healthy diet should be a process you enjoy every day, not something you dread.

Sure, we need to make some sacrifices, but we shouldn't go to other extremes where a mind-numbing overhaul of diet and training simply can't be sustained in the long term.

It might have taken me 18 years of experimenting with countless training methods and diet plans, and reading a ridiculous amount of fitness articles and books.

You don't need all that hassle because what's in this book WORKS. It keeps me strong, in great shape, and most importantly, in great health. I've seen clients and close friends achieve fantastic results by applying the same tactics.

Know what? This is effectively just another "how to" book…and there are plenty of them out there. What's more important is whether or not you DO the "how to".

Are you going to skip planning out your workouts in advance because you've got better things to do? Are you going to do the exercises - but give squats a miss because you've never really like doing them?

If so, then you might aswell not bother at all. Not trying to lecture you. This entire book is just friendly advice based on experience, experimentation and education. But I've got to underline that this is all about <u>action</u>.

If you want to build muscle, lose fat and feel strong, healthy and happy then you've got to keep showing up. You've got to be disciplined and back all your efforts up with the right mindset.

The first step in achieving that mindset firm focus is proper preparation and setting clear, defined goals. Chapter 2 shows you how to do this effectively – which naturally boosts your motivation levels and makes it much less likely you'll go off track.

There are then 10 compound exercises, with some isolation moves, to focus on. Master these and then you'll have weight training mastered. These are the biggest, best, and most effective exercises for developing muscle.

Your strength will go through the roof, you'll make gains you never expected, and you'll enjoy the process.

But it's all about sticking with the programme long enough – and not forgetting the other important ingredients, which include:

- Progressively overloading the muscles using The 3,6,9 Principle.

- Adding variety to your training routine to keep shocking the muscles into growth.

- Switching to a different training system every 4-6 weeks.

- Following a healthy whole foods diet – and paying more attention to sufficient calories rather than crazy amounts of protein.

- ….and giving yourself the edge with 'The Essentials' supplements.

These are just a handful of some of the key lessons. I've also included the checklist at the end of each chapter so it's easy for you to revisit the most important pieces of information - without having to read everything again.

We all want to be in the best shape possible. There are many thousands of people telling us many thousands of ways of achieving this.

When I first started weight training aged 16 I saw a small ad in FHM magazine for a book that promised the secret to building serious muscle. Desperate to transform my embarrassingly skinny physique, I sent £20 in the mail to buy it.

The next week a black and white book arrived at my house. I'll sum up the book's "secret to building serious muscle": lift weights, make sure those weights are heavy…and drink lots of milk!

Not everything I was expecting, and gulping gallons of milk was a bad idea. But do you know what? It was money well spent because it included most of the compound exercises I'm obsessed with now, and it taught me to go as heavy as possible.

I've shared that same advice here, but there was so much more to learn. I delved deeper into training, nutrition, recovery, supplements etc over the next 18 years, and have now passed on what I consider the best strategies and tools for success in building muscle and burning fat.

Strength Training Program 101 doesn't follow the typical advice being spewed out by gym Meatheads, or a large chunk of the health and fitness industry.

That's intentional. Their way is not the only way to develop the strong, lean, athletic physique you want. This approach can also be maintained more easily with just three or four weight training sessions per week.

Training 5,6,7 days per week is unnecessary and can be counter-productive. This way is effective, efficient and crucially gives your body the rest periods it needs for proper recovery and growth.

If you've tried everything to get in great shape before and got nowhere then this can be your ticket to success. Or if you're just starting out in lifting weights then you've probably saved yourself many months and years of trying to figure out the best way to get results.

Forget everyone else. This is all about becoming a stronger, healthier, better version of you.

I created this book to help other people transform their body, health and to receive the multiple benefits I have from strength training over the years. I want you to get the most out of it…that's why I've created a special bonus e-book with photo demonstrations of me performing every exercise.

This will help anyone who is less experienced or is just not familiar with some of the exercises I mentioned earlier. You can download it for FREE online at: www.weighttrainingistheway.com/exercise-demos

All the best going forward, my fellow Non-Meathead friend.

Marc McLean.

P.S.....

I hope you enjoyed this book and got some real value from it. I'd really appreciate it if you quickly jumped over to Amazon and left me a book review.

The '4 Keys' To Getting In The Best Shape Of Your Life

Do you get really enthusiastic about finally getting rid of the belly fat and developing muscle, make a little progress…but then end up back at square one?

Do you struggle to find motivation for exercise…and sometimes simply get bored with it all?

Do you get frustrated when you look in the mirror and see zero changes to your bodyshape despite working hard for weeks, maybe even months?

It ain't your fault. Training hard and eating well are only part of the equation. What most people don't realise is that getting these two factors right will only get you so far.

In my experience as a strength training coach, I've found that men and women only reach a certain level because they don't know have the '4 Keys' that are essential to health and fitness success.

Do you realise that you may actually be sabotaging your hard efforts to achieve your health and fitness goals - without even realising it?

I'd love to reveal these 4 keys to you and help you blitz bodyfat, develop lean muscle, and become strong as hell!

As a thank you for buying this book, I've created a mini video series titled **"The 4 Keys To Getting In The Best Shape Of Your Life"** that you can access for **FREE**.

These short video lessons cover each of these 4 keys that are essential for not only transforming your mind, body and health, but ensuring you stay that way too!

To access the mini video series online visit:
www.getleanandstrong.com/four-keys

About the author

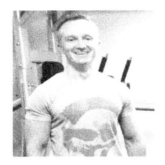

Marc McLean is a 34 year old online personal training and nutrition coach from Loch Lomond in Scotland. He owns Weight Training Is The Way and is a health and fitness writer for leading websites including The Good Men Project, Mind Body Green, and Healthgreatness.com

Marc loves...climbing Munros (aka the biggest hills) in Scotland, peanut butter, amazing scenery, the Rocky movies, lifting heavy things, blueberries, Daft Punk, watching tennis, travelling and laughing. Not in that particular order.

Marc hates...bad manners, funerals, cardio, and all drivers who don't indicate.

You can connect with Marc here:

Email: marc@weighttrainingistheway.com

Website: www.weighttrainingistheway.com

Facebook: www.facebook.com/weighttrainingistheway

Instagram: www.instagram.com/weight_training_is_the_way

Printed in Great Britain
by Amazon